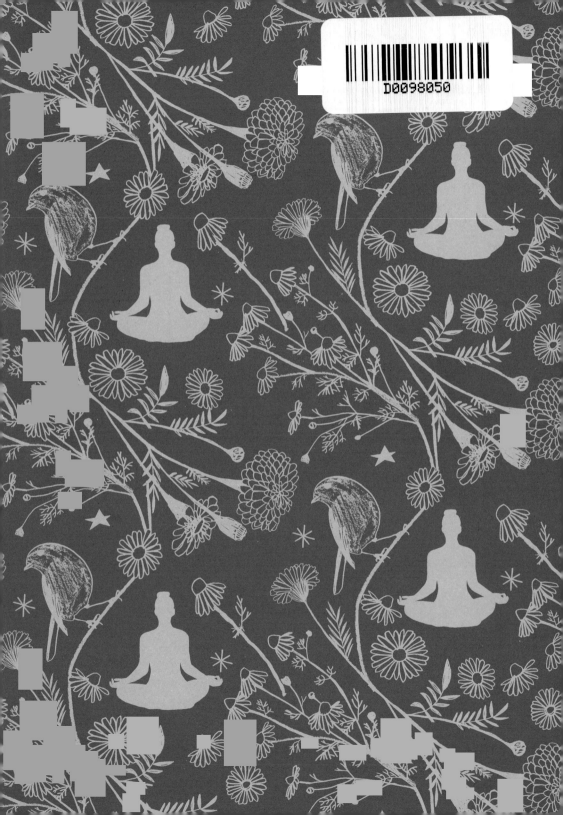

D0098050

wellness
WITCH

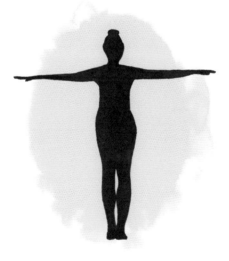

wellness WITCH

Healing Potions, Soothing Spells,
and Empowering Rituals
for Magical Self-Care

NIKKI VAN DE CAR

Illustrations by ANISA MAKHOUL

RUNNING PRESS
PHILADELPHIA

Note: The information in this book is true and complete to the best of our knowledge. This book is intended only as an informative guide for those wishing to know more about herbal remedies. In no way is this book intended to replace, countermand, or conflict with the advice given to you by your own physician. The ultimate decision concerning care should be made between you and your doctor. We strongly recommend you follow his or her advice. Information in this book is general and is offered with no guarantees on the part of the authors or Running Press. The authors and publisher disclaim all liability in connection with the use of this book.

Recipes adapted from Emily of Layers of Happiness,
Amy of She Wears Many Hats, Deb Perelman of Smitten Kitchen.

Copyright © 2019 by Nikki Van De Car
Illustrations copyright © 2019 by Anisa Makhoul
Cover copyright © 2019 by Hachette Book Group, Inc.

Hachette Book Group supports the right to free expression and the value of copyright. The purpose of copyright is to encourage writers and artists to produce the creative works that enrich our culture.

The scanning, uploading, and distribution of this book without permission is a theft of the author's intellectual property. If you would like permission to use material from the book (other than for review purposes), please contact permissions@hbgusa.com. Thank you for your support of the author's rights.

Running Press
Hachette Book Group
1290 Avenue of the Americas, New York, NY 10104
www.runningpress.com
@Running_Press

Printed in China
First Edition: September 2019

Published by Running Press, an imprint of Perseus Books, LLC, a subsidiary of Hachette Book Group, Inc. The Running Press name and logo is a trademark of the Hachette Book Group.

The Hachette Speakers Bureau provides a wide range of authors for speaking events. To find out more, go to www.hachettespeakersbureau.com or call (866) 376-6591.

The publisher is not responsible for websites (or their content) that are not owned by the publisher.

Print book cover and interior design by Susan Van Horn.

Library of Congress Control Number: 2019937274

ISBNs: 978-0-7624-6734-1 (hardcover), 978-0-7624-6732-7 (ebook)

1010

10 9 8 7 6 5 4 3 2 1

contents

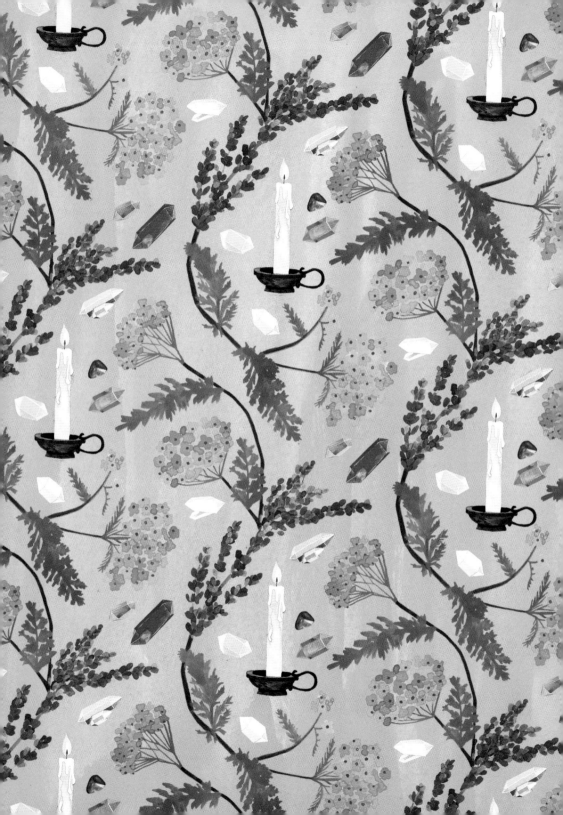

INTRODUCTION

The simplest and, therefore, often the most powerful form of witchcraft is what we do ourselves, for ourselves. Today's wellness witch is part of a long and honored tradition of invoking the natural world, personal creativity, healing, and the power of the feminine. This kind of magic transmutes surviving into thriving and basic health into true wellness and personal power.

Becoming a wellness witch can begin with something as simple as intention—as, indeed, all magic does. When preparing a meal, direct your thoughts to the sustenance it brings with gratitude for the life you take from your food. Then, go a step further and season with herbs that enhance your intention—whether for healing, prosperity, love, or psychic power. Remember always that your body is a temple, the vessel through which you live your life. Use your spirit's connection with your physical self to enhance the whole through something as simple as a gentle balm or even a powerful essential oil potion. And make your home, your hearth, into a place that lifts you up, soothing and inspiring you.

The concoctions, teas, rituals, and spells in this book are merely a jumping-off point, a way for you to begin your wellness magic practice and then expand into creating and refining it for yourself. For instance, most potions here include instructions on methods of stirring, either clockwise or counterclockwise. The choice you make depends on the *kind* of potion you're producing. If it's a healing potion, then you want to harness the power of the sun by following its path clockwise as your stir to invite that energy into your work. On the other hand, if you're expanding your awareness into the mysterious, the unknown, and the unseen, stirring counterclockwise or widdershins helps fulfill that intention.

Along those same lines, gathering fresh herbs by moonlight or sunlight, or charging dried herbs thereby, follows a similar pattern. Moonlight evokes femininity and mystery; it allows you to see into the depths of the soul. Sunlight, on the other hand, invites warmth and healing, and often a kind of childlike joy. But if you want to work your spell at a different time of the month or sunlight or moonlight isn't available to you for whatever reason, make your own adjustments based on what you will learn here and follow your own instincts. A candle, a lamp, a stone, or even a whispered spell can produce the same results as drawing on the power of the celestial bodies—as always, it is about intention.

The power, the *magic*, that comes from making something yourself, free of harmful chemicals and imbued with mystical essence, and the knowledge that you can create everything you need or want . . . is undeniable. By calling on the traditions and expertise of women who have come before us and merging it with our own intuition and creativity, we can bring peace, power, and everyday magic into our lives. Wellness magic is not just something you *do*; it's a way of life.

THE GARDEN

A wellness witch relies on her garden. She grows her herbs with care and intention, harvests them at the right time, and dries them in bundles that hang around her hearth and home.

That home, of course, will vary from witch to witch. We can't all live in a cottage in the woods. But a tiny studio apartment or even just the corner of a bedroom can be enchanting—as can its garden. The size and location are meaningless, for it's the intention of the gardener that matters.

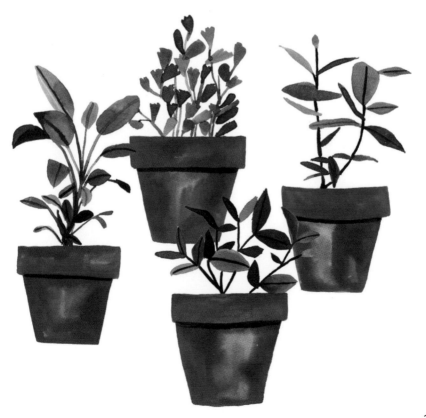

In a plot of earth or a small window box, cultivate any combination of the following commonly used herbs:

BLUE VERVAIN: Vervain should be allowed to flower for a few days before it is collected. Both the leaves and the flowers should be harvested; trim the vervain as you would thyme, and pinch off the flowers to dry separately as you would with marigold or chamomile.

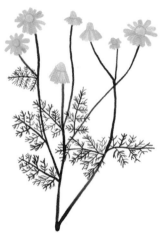

CHAMOMILE: The flower is the most beneficial part of this plant, and you'll want to wait to harvest it until it is at its peak—which tends to vary from blossom to blossom. When the sun is high in the sky in the late morning, go through your chamomile looking for a blossom that is *just about* to open. Pinch it off at the base and leave it to dry in a woven basket, adding more flowers to your collection throughout the summer. Be sure to allow a few blossoms to go to seed so that your chamomile will continue on next year.

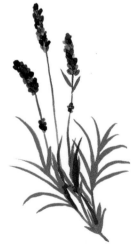

LAVENDER: Allow your lavender to come into full bloom, then trim the stem three inches or so below the flowers, using scissors or a harvesting knife. Do this in the early morning, before the dew has dried. Gather the stems into a bundle and hang this upside down to dry.

LEMON BALM: Lemon balm can be used fresh, a few leaves at a time, or it can be harvested by cutting the stem two inches above the soil before it begins to flower. Bundle and hang upside down to dry.

MARIGOLD: Calendula, or marigold, will thank you for each flower you take, pushing to give you more. Cut the stem of each flower head at the base of the leaves, harvesting in the early morning before the dew begins to evaporate. Pinch off each flower and allow it to dry in a basket out of direct sunlight. This may take longer than you expect—give it two weeks, just to be safe. Leave a few seeds for next season, of course!

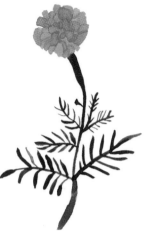

MINT: Use fresh leaves as often as possible, but when your mint starts to get unruly, cut it down to one inch above the ground just before it flowers. Tie the stems, and hang them upside down to dry or freeze them.

MUGWORT: Mugwort should be harvested just as the plant begins to flower, before the blooms open completely. Remove the leaves and flower heads and dry them separately on paper-lined trays; do not hang dry.

MULLEIN: Use mullein fresh, or dry just a few leaves at a time on a cloth for its first year. By the second year the plant will be hardy enough to harvest the leaves by cutting the thickest stems close to the base of the stalk and bundling and drying them as with sage. You can also harvest and dry the flowers and buds for similar use.

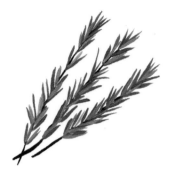

ROSEMARY: You can use fresh sprigs throughout most of the year, as rosemary is fairly hardy even in cold weather. To harvest, collect the sprigs about three inches from the top of the plant, just as they start to bloom. Tie a bundle and hang it upside down to dry.

SAGE: Use fresh sage a few leaves at a time. To harvest for drying, take the maturest stems just before they go to seed, cutting them right down at the base of the plant. Lay your stems in the same direction and tie them tightly together with string. Hang your bundle upside down to dry for at least a week.

THYME: Thyme can always be used fresh, but grows so rapidly that harvesting is often a necessity. Harvest your thyme midmorning by cutting near the base of the plant just below a new branch filled with healthy leaves. Bundle this up and hang it to dry.

YARROW: Harvest your yarrow after the flowers are in full bloom, cutting the entire stem halfway down the plant. Bundle your stems and dry them hanging upside down out of direct sunlight.

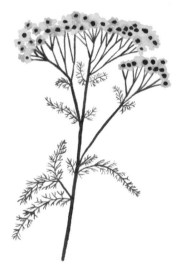

THE CUPBOARD

Just as there are plants that you'll return to again and again, there are several items that are always useful to have on hand. You don't need a cauldron, but a decent-size pot is a good idea—in fact, you'll need two, since you don't want to make candles and poultices in the same saucepan you use to brew tea. On the other hand, you really only need one mortar and pestle, since the herbs you'll be employing are edible. You'll need a good selection of jars, spray bottles, and containers, including some of those dark blue or brown glass bottles for storing tinctures and essential oil blends.

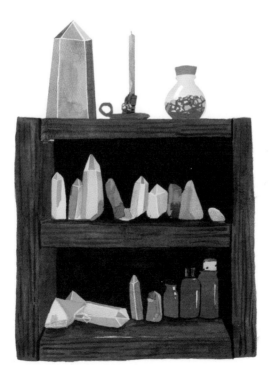

crystals

There are a *lot* of powerful crystals out there, and the study and practice of determining which ones work best for you are part of your growth as a witch. However, these stones are a good place to start:

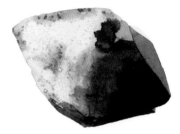

AMETHYST: This stone activates your crown chakra, connecting you with the mystical unknown. Amethyst aids in meditation, calm, and tranquility and relieves headaches.

AQUAMARINE: This gem opens your throat chakra, aiding you in expression of your personal truth, and reduces fear and tension.

CALCITE: Calcite amplifies your energies, allowing you to communicate with the spiritual world.

CLEAR QUARTZ: You could limit your collection to clear quartz alone, if you wanted, because clear quartz can be programmed to serve whatever function you require of it. To do this, simply hold the crystal and focus your intentions. If you leave clear quartz as is, it will serve as a general healing stone.

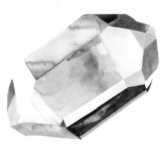

HEMATITE: This is a protective stone, one that will ground you and close your aura to negative energies.

LAPIS LAZULI: A powerful stone of focus, it will aid in meditation.

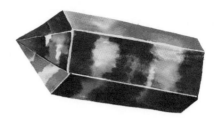

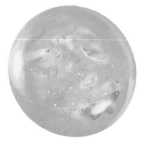

OPAL: Opal is another energy amplifier and will enhance any mystical practices by inviting creativity.

Your crystals will need to be cleared and charged every so often, depending on how regularly you use them. Clear your stones with wild running water, such as a stream or rain, or by soaking them in salt water or smudging them with sage.

Activating a crystal can be as simple as holding the stone while focusing on your intention for it, but if you have a little more time, you can perform the following ritual.

Stand in pure light—sunlight if you're looking for clarity, moonlight if you're looking for mystery—and cup your crystal in your hands so that the light shines upon it. Set your intention for the stone, speaking it aloud or in your mind, and then hold the stone to your heart as you bow your head and give thanks.

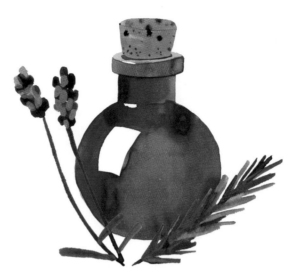

essential oils

Essential oils are, well, essential! They are the purest distillation of the healing plants you will use—a drop of spearmint essential oil is more powerful than a fresh leaf. Again, there are a *lot* of them out there, from a wide variety of sources that can vary in quality. For the most part, purchase what you can afford; there's no need to plunk down fifty dollars for a tiny bottle of frankincense oil. Look for therapeutic-grade oil, but don't stress about how highly rated it is, as there's no governing body managing such claims. Make sure your oil is pure—100 percent undiluted—and definitely don't drink it. Even essential oils made from herbs we normally eat, like sage or thyme, can be toxic because they are so very intense. Some essential oils are so strong that they are best diluted with a carrier oil like olive or almond oil before they are used directly on your skin.

You'll want to investigate which essential oils work best for you, depending on your personal preference, but here are a few to get you started:

CHAMOMILE: This gentle oil is useful for skin care—it's safe to apply directly on your skin—bugbites, and inducing calm.

CLOVE: This surprisingly powerful oil is good for respiratory and digestive health, as a disinfectant, and as an aphrodisiac.

GINGER: Ginger is warming, energetic, and helpful in reducing joint pain.

LAVENDER: The ultimate in soothing and relaxing essential oils, lavender is safe to apply to the skin and can be used to reduce headaches, help with sleep, clean, and restore emotional balance.

LEMON: It's not such a great idea to use lemon oil directly on your skin, as it can cause a sunburn, but its healing, disinfecting, and energizing properties can work wonders when blended with a carrier oil.

PEPPERMINT: Peppermint provides a welcome lift, both in your respiratory system and in your heart and mind.

ROSE: Properly diluted with a carrier oil, rose is as good for your skin as it is for your heart. It gives a sense of calm optimism.

SWEET ORANGE: This is the happiest of all essential oils. It calms inflammation and soothes allergies, but more than anything, it provides comfort and a sense of well-being.

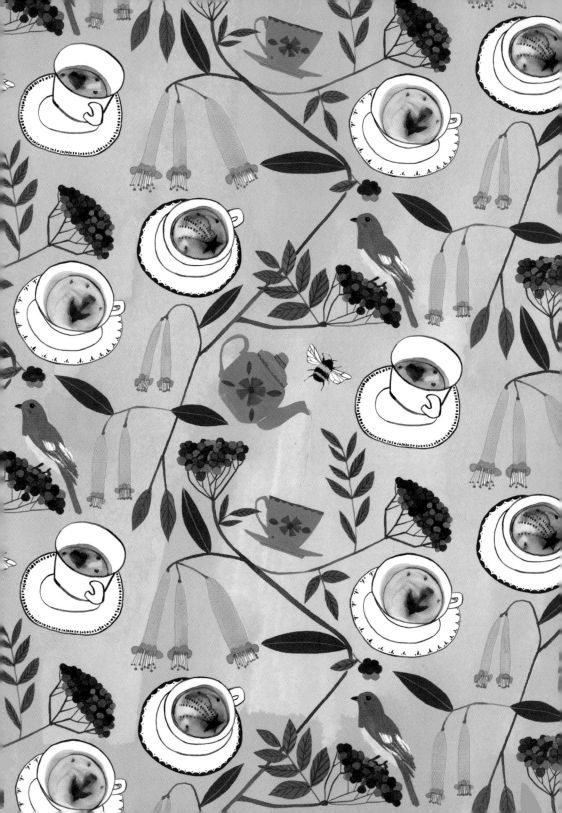

THe
INTERNaL

All the work we do in this world starts from within, and magic is no exception. In order to become truly powerful, we must grow our own personal strength. This section features rituals, spells, and recipes that all work toward the same goal: increasing your personal power. In this and all sections, we start with healing, move on to soothing, and finally reach empowering—for it is only when we are healed, calm, and open that we can find the source of our power. Be aware: you'll be drinking A LOT of tea.

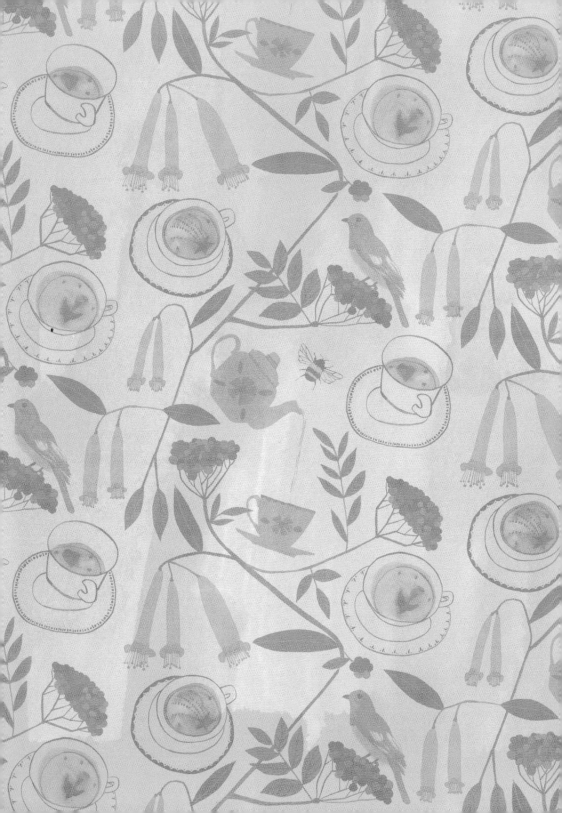

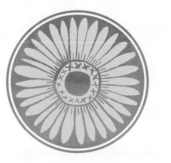

HEALING

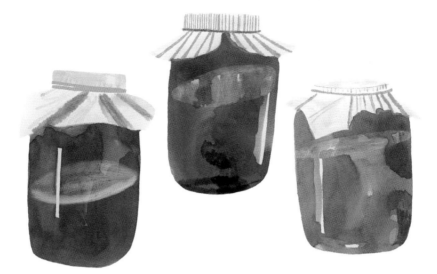

KOMBUCHA

MOST OF US WOULD-BE WELLNESS WITCHES HAVE ENJOYED our fair share of kombucha. After all, kombucha has been around for thousands of years, fermenting in the kitchens of women for whom magic was just a part of daily life. Dating back to at least 250 BC this "tea fungus" was highly prized for its friendly digestive properties.

Today, plunking down four dollars for a delicious, healthy beverage—it's basically soda that's good for you!—seems perfectly reasonable until you consider that there is another option. This perhaps requires a bit more work in the beginning, but it's entirely worth it. Making your own kombucha is a creative, thrifty, and quite fun endeavor—and it's much less intimidating than it may seem at first.

Start off by purchasing one of those four-dollar bottles. You'll want to look for one that's a little long in the tooth, with a fair amount of material floating around the bottom. In the past, perhaps, you might have avoided those bottles—but that gunk is the good stuff, the start of your scoby.

Working with the scoby is likely going to be the most intimidating part of your kombucha making . . . some even find it downright scary. Scoby is a shortened way of saying a symbiotic culture of bacteria and yeast, and this rubbery, slimy disc is a literal colony of life, imbuing your sweet tea with nutrients and friendly microbes. While it does appear, at first, to be a little gross, there's something very tender and magical about the ability to hold an entire universe in your hands.

growing a scoby

Enjoy all but half a cup of that bottled kombucha, saving the solids for your scoby. Bring seven cups of water to a boil, and stir in half a cup of white sugar until it is dissolved. Dip four bags of plain black tea into your sugar water and allow it to steep until your tea has cooled to room temperature, at which point you can remove the bags.

Pour the reserved half cup of kombucha and the room temperature tea into a big jar. Cover the jar with a cloth secured with a rubber band, and allow the mixture to rest in a dark place for three to four weeks. During this time, your scoby will grow from those murky bits into a rubbery disk that fits the top of your jar, with perhaps some strings dangling from the bottom.

making the kombucha

You'll have to toss all but half a cup of that original batch of kombucha; the growing scoby will have consumed all the sugar and it will taste more or less like vinegar. You can use the liquid to clean your windows and counters, though—a wellness witch is nothing if not resourceful!

But the principle for your next batch is basically the same; brew another seven cups of strong, sweet tea. (You can experiment with caffeine-free kombucha once your scoby is big and strong; for the first few batches, stick with plain black tea.) Let the tea cool and add it to your scoby jar and the half cup of your original kombucha. This time, it will only need to rest for seven to ten days.

When that time is up, brew *another* seven cups of strong, sweet tea and let it cool. Transfer the scoby to a second large jar along with half a cup of its kombucha. Add the new sweet tea and cover and store for another seven to ten days to begin your next batch.

The rest of the kombucha is nearly ready to drink! Add some fresh fruit, ginger, turmeric, herbs—whatever seems tasty and is fresh and available—and cover your jar with its lid. Refrigerate for a day or two, allowing the carbonation to really set in. And then—enjoy!

scoby health

Once you've been continuously brewing your kombucha in this fashion for a while, you'll notice your scoby getting a little thick. This will cause your kombucha to start tasting more vinegary. Simply peel off a few layers of the scoby and either toss them or give them to a fellow witch looking to start her own batch.

You'll want to keep an eye on your scoby; they can occasionally develop mold or some kind of imbalance. Black marks or fuzzy spots mean your scoby needs to be tossed—but it's simple enough to grow a new one.

AYURVEDIC TEA

⊱──o──⊰

THE SYSTEM OF AYURVEDA WAS DEVELOPED IN INDIA THOUSANDS of years ago; the term literally means "the science of life." The tradition is based on the principle that the mind and body are deeply connected, and therefore, the mind—if properly nourished and empowered—can heal the body. You can nourish your mind through meditation, a balance of rest and exercise since the relationship between the body and the mind is symbiotic, and the use of specific herbal remedies. Ayurvedic tradition includes thousands of herbs; this tea uses some that specifically address aligning the mind with the body to reduce stress and tension:

- Ashwaganda
- Brahmi or gotu kola
- Jatamansi or spikenard

These three herbs are both calming and balancing: Ashwaganda will reduce the stress hormone cortisol in your brain. Brahmi or gotu kola helps drain the brain of toxins. And jatamansi, also known as spikenard, acts as a calming antidepressant. These botanicals are all available for order online, or you can find them at health food stores.

None of these herbs, however, taste that good. You may choose to take them as a supplement, but they can be consumed as a tea as long as they are balanced with other equally healing, but tastier, plants—which are generally also easier to find:

- Cinnamon
- Cardamom
- Ginger root
- Holy basil
- Clove
- Turmeric

Cinnamon enhances brain function, turmeric reduces inflammation, and holy basil is deeply calming. Cardamom, clove, and ginger root enhance circulation and digestion—their inclusion in your tea will therefore help your body process the other beneficial herbs.

You can make a tea using any combination of the above, choosing whatever is most readily available to you! You'll want to keep your ingredients as fresh and close to whole as possible and use a 1:2 ratio when you're planning your tea: use half as many not-so-great-tasting herbs as more fragrant herbs.

If you're using ginger, slice the root up first, though there's no need to peel it. Add all your ingredients to a mortar and, using your pestle, crush them together, splitting open your cardamom pods and breaking down your cinnamon sticks. Use the wetness of the ginger to bring life to any dried herbs you have in your mixture. You'll want about ½ cup of blended herbs in total. Take notes about what you use and in which quantities; every body and every mind is unique and will react differently to these ingredients, so you'll want to pay attention and adjust your recipe until you've found the perfect blend for you.

Bring two quarts of water to a boil. With intention, add your chosen ingredients and stir clockwise for clarity. Lower the heat to a simmer, cover, and let your tea brew for at least half an hour, or as long as two or three hours.

Pour your tea through a strainer or cheesecloth into a jar or pitcher. It can be enjoyed both hot and cold and is generally sweetened with a little honey and milk (for antibacterial and general deliciousness purposes, but also because both honey and milk are traditional offerings to various deities).

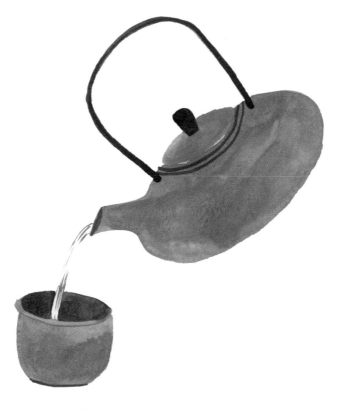

TEA RITUAL

MANY CULTURES IN ASIA PRACTICE TEA CEREMONIES. IN CHINA the act of making tea for someone else is inscribed with meaning—to show respect, gratitude, or even apology—while in Japan the ceremony begins with a ritual purification and everything from examining the tea cup to where you place your lips to take your first sip is done with very specific intention.

Your own tea ritual can be just as specific, or it can be looser, allowing the experiences of the day to inform the choices you make. Either way, the act of drinking a cup of tea can be a form of magic—something much more meaningful than a simple beverage you keep next to your computer while you work—although it can certainly be that, too. The *kind* of tea you drink matters, as different teas provoke different responses in your body. Ayurvedic tradition teaches us that our minds have a profound effect on our bodies—so it is only logical that imbuing our tea with meaning through the practice of ritual will enhance the effects of that tea, making it even more powerful.

Before you brew a cup of tea, wash your face and hands. Come into your ritual with a clean slate, so to speak. Put your water on to boil, whether you are using a tea kettle, an electric kettle, or a simple pot of water—it doesn't matter. While the water is heating, close your eyes and take three deep, cleansing breaths.

Choose your mug with care. This may seem silly, but it does matter. Do you want something comforting, like the mug you've had since you were a child? Do you want something beautiful and inspiring, like a china teacup? Do you want the mug with the silly slogan or one that references a television show you love? We all have associations with the *things* in our lives; choose an association that feels right for this cup of tea, today.

When your water is boiling, turn it off. Allow it rest until the bubbles have subsided. Ready your tea strainer. Slowly, with a steady stream of water approximately six inches above the brim, fill your cup with water. Allow it to steep for the recommended period—if you like, use this time for meditation, deep breathing, or even simple daydreaming.

When your tea is ready, remove the strainer and bring the cup to your face. Close your eyes. Inhale deeply three times. Focus your intention for this cup of tea and what it will bring you. Then, take your first sip.

If you like, continue drinking with intention and contemplation, focusing on your experience in the moment. But you can also at this point go sit down on the couch with a good book, call up a friend you haven't talked to in a while, or anything that feels equally nourishing to your spirit.

BROKEN HEART BREAD

WE HAVE ALL HAD OUR HEARTS BROKEN. WHETHER FROM a failed romance, a bereavement, a fight with a loved one, or a dream unfulfilled—we all suffer those feelings of despair. And though we all know they are temporary, they don't *feel* temporary at the time. We feel sadness, anger, hurt—all emotions we usually try to avoid.

But sometimes, the only way through those emotions is to get close to them, to immerse ourselves in them. We don't always allow ourselves to truly feel our anger, and we try to turn away from our own sadness. For most of us, this doesn't really work and instead leaves us simmering in those emotions for longer than we need to.

Getting close to traditionally negative emotions isn't easy, though. You have to decide to do it, to take action. The ritual of making and eating this bread can help with that.

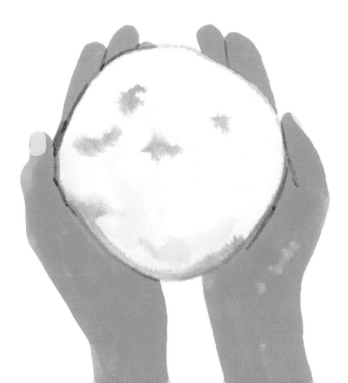

½ teaspoon
dried marjoram

½ teaspoon
dried sage

½ teaspoon dried
garlic powder

1½ teaspoons
kosher salt

1½ cups very
warm water

1½ teaspoons honey

1½ teaspoons active
dry yeast

3 cups bread flour
+ a little more for
kneading

1½ tablespoons
olive oil

Begin by mixing your herbs together with your salt. Grind them in your mortar and pestle, breaking them down and integrating them with one another. Remind yourself that marjoram is for grief, sage is for clarity, garlic is for protection. The salt is for protection, purification, and blessing and will bind all the components together.

Put the warm water in a large bowl. Stir in your honey, and then sprinkle the mixture with yeast. Allow the yeast five minutes to activate. During this time, add your herbs to the flour, making sure they are mixed in evenly. Stir the flour mixture into the yeasty water using a wooden spoon. Add the olive oil. Stir twenty-one times (seven and three are both very powerful numbers) in a clockwise direction to allow you time to see your own emotions.

Cover your bowl with a dishcloth and allow it to rest for one and a half hours, or until it has doubled in size. While the dough is rising, write in your journal. Meditate. Go for a run. Do whatever allows you to clear your mind, but get close to your emotions. When the hour and a half is up, sprinkle some flour on your counter or tabletop, and lift the dough out of the bowl, placing it onto your flour. It will be fluffy and sticky. Knead your dough seven times—and put your heart into this. With each fold and press of your fist into the dough, release any anger, any sadness, any hurt. Punch those feelings into the dough. When you're done, gently and lovingly fold your dough into a nice round shape and carefully place it on a baking sheet covered in parchment paper.

Leave your dough on the counter and let it rise for another hour. Spend that time in an intentional, healing way. Heat your oven to 450 degrees, and let the dough continue to rise for another half hour. Just before putting it into the oven, flick the loaf with water three times. Bake for twenty-five to thirty minutes, or until the bread sounds hollow when knocked.

When it's done, remove your bread from the oven and let it rest on a cooling rack for five minutes so the bottom remains firm. Slice thickly, and eat warm, spread with butter and honey. You have put your heart into this bread—now take it back into yourself, for it is yours, and it is whole.

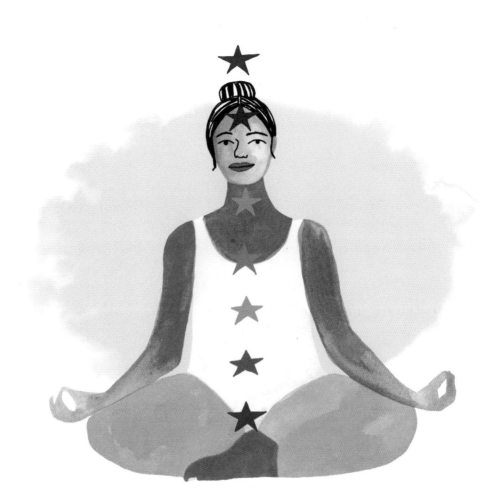

CRYSTAL CHAKRA RITUAL

THIS RITUAL IS FOCUSED AROUND OPENING YOUR CHAKRAS, the seven points of energy in your body. They each serve different functions, and bringing them all into balance keeps *you* in balance.

★ **MULADHARA, THE ROOT CHAKRA:** Located at the base of the spine, this is our chakra of instinct, safety, and our connection with the earth. It responds to the color red and stones associated with safety, so choose hematite, red jasper, or garnet for your root chakra.

★ **SVADHISTHANA, THE SACRAL CHAKRA:** This chakra is the center of our creativity and sexuality. It is the source of our passion and our pleasure. It responds to orange stones like citrine or carnelian, but also to moonstone, which represents our feminine connection to mystery and fertility.

★ **MANIPURA, THE SOLAR PLEXUS CHAKRA:** This is our source of strength and our will. Bright as the sun, manipura responds to yellow jasper, pyrite, or the powerful tigereye.

★ **ANAHATA, THE HEART CHAKRA:** The central chakra, and arguably the most important, is your source and your receptor for love of all kinds—romantic love, friendship, self-love, and love of the world. Anahata is traditionally green-colored and responds to malachite, but our cultural associations with rose quartz make it a natural choice as well.

★ **VISHUDDHA, THE THROAT CHAKRA:** This is the connection to your power to communicate and send your power out beyond yourself. Its color is light blue, like aquamarine or turquoise.

★ **AJNA, THE THIRD EYE CHAKRA:** This is the chakra of wisdom, of the ability to see clearly and deeply. Its indigo nature responds best to stones like lapis lazuli and azurite.

★ **SAHASRARA, THE CROWN CHAKRA:** Sahasrara connects you with the mystical power of the universe, with all that is unknown but felt, unseen but present. This deep purple chakra responds best to amethyst or to clear bright stones like clear quartz or selenite.

Begin by allowing yourself time, peace, and quiet. Find a ritual space that works for you—this can be your bedroom, the floor, a patch of grass, or anywhere you can lie flat—but make sure it feels calm and free of negative energy. If you're surrounded by work left undone, unfolded laundry, stacks of bills, and the like, that energy will invade you as you open yourself up. Give yourself as pure and healing a space as you can. Extend this by lighting candles, burning sage, or playing gentle music—follow your instincts here! Gather, cleanse and program your stones, infusing them with your intention. Set a timer for fifteen or twenty minutes.

Lie flat and ready the crystals for placement. Beginning at the crown chakra, hold your stone to the top of your head for the space of a long breath, then place it an inch or so above your head, on the floor. Moving to the third eye chakra, place your stone right on your third eye. Place your throat, heart, and solar plexus chakra stones at their appropriate locations, and position your sacral chakra stone just below your navel. Hold your root chakra stone in the open palm of your nondominant hand.

Lie flat, breathing deeply and evenly, as you allow the crystals to come into resonance with your chakras and with each other. You may feel your body and your emotions responding to certain chakras, as you experience heat, vibrations, or even emotional release. Allow it all.

When your timer goes off, don't get up right away. Come back to your body, to your present moment, but do it slowly, allowing yourself to make the journey with ease and care. Remove your stones in the reverse order that you placed them. Take one last deep breath and release it before opening your eyes.

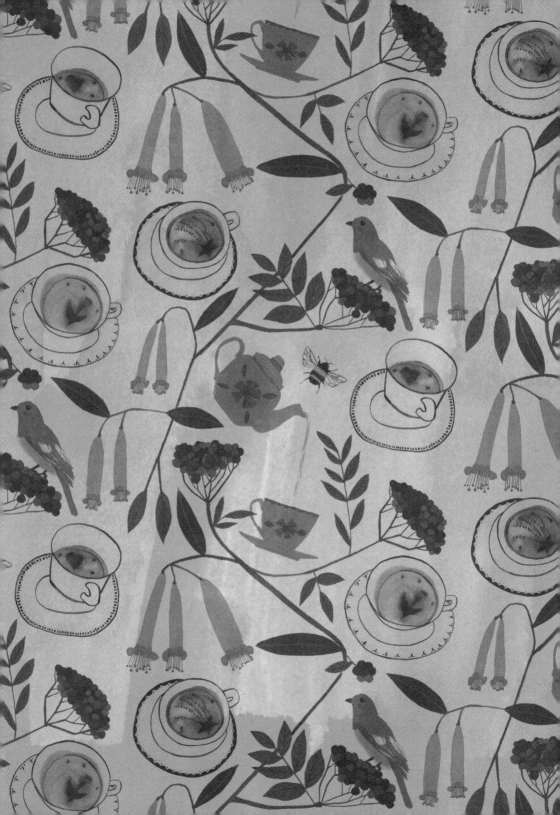

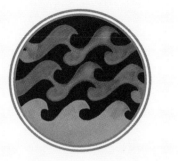

SOOTHING

LAVENDER CHAMOMILE CUPCAKES

CUPCAKES SOOTHE THE SOUL. THEY ARE DAINTY, PRETTY LITTLE things, and they warm our hearts and make us smile.

That in and of itself is deeply magical—and deeply important. The inherent magic of pleasure—whether it's a glass of wine, or rolling down a hill, or getting a massage—is that we are doing something simply because it brings us joy. That is enough—and better yet, it is valuable for its own sake, so that we can experience the magical bliss of life. Yes, cupcakes contain butter . . . and sugar . . . and white flour! These things can be *celebrated* and indulged in deeply and mindfully. While substantive, these cupcakes are not overly sweet. They are a gift we give ourselves and anyone else who might be in need of them.

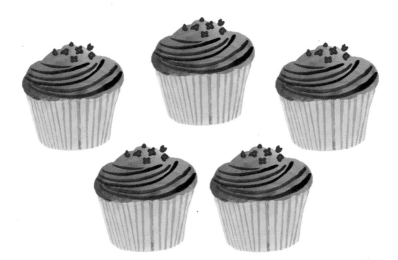

cake

1 teaspoon dried chamomile

1 teaspoon alcohol-based vanilla extract

2 cups flour

2 teaspoons baking powder

½ teaspoon salt

1 cup milk

½ cup butter, at room temperature

¾ cup sugar

2 eggs

The day before you plan to make these cupcakes, grind your chamomile into a fine powder using your mortar and pestle. Sprinkle your vanilla extract over the chamomile (the alcohol will help the chamomile flavor infuse the final cupcake). Pour this into a small jar or other closed container, and allow your mixture to steep overnight. If you can, place it in a location where the morning light will warm it slightly, surrounded by moonstone and amethyst.

When you're ready to make your cupcakes, begin by preheating your oven to 375 degrees. Line your muffin tin with papers. Mix your flour, baking powder, and salt together using a wooden spoon, stirring in a clockwise direction. Pour your chamomile-vanilla solution into the measuring cup containing your milk.

Using an electric or stand mixer, begin blending your butter and sugar together at medium speed until it is light and fluffy—usually three to five minutes. Beat in your eggs one at a time. Then, add half a cup of the flour mixture and blend at low speed. Add a quarter cup of your milk mixture and blend. Alternate in this fashion until all the ingredients are well-mixed.

Pour your batter into the prepared muffin tin and bake for eighteen minutes, or until the cupcakes are golden brown. Remove the cupcakes from the tin and allow them to cool while you make the frosting.

frosting

2 cups powdered sugar

⅓ cup hot water

3 tablespoons fresh or dried lavender flowers

2 large egg whites, room temperature

¼ teaspoon salt

½ teaspoon cream of tartar

Begin by making a lavender simple syrup. Whisk together your powdered sugar, hot water, and lavender in a saucepan and raise the heat until it comes to a boil. Allow your mixture to boil for one minute, whisking constantly, and then remove the pan from the heat. Strain out the lavender and set aside for a moment.

Using a clean and completely dry electric or stand mixer, mix the egg whites together with the salt and cream of tartar at high speed. Slowly pour in the hot simple syrup in a small stream. When it has all been added, continue to beat at a high speed until a nice, spreadable consistency has been reached.

By now the cupcakes should be cool enough to frost, but double-check them just in case. Spread the frosting generously, and decorate with the lavender you set aside or chamomile flowers if you have them. Share with friends and loved ones, but make sure to eat just one by yourself, sitting with a cup of tea, and allow yourself the pleasure of this sweet, soothing gift.

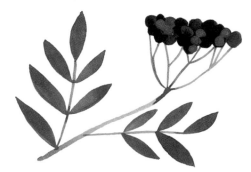

ELDERBERRY SYRUP

THIS RECIPE IS ANCIENT—AND AS EFFICACIOUS AS EVER. Lemon and honey are a time-honored healing combination, as their vitamin C and antibacterial effects, respectively, blend together so soothingly. Mullein and yarrow both tend to coughs, sore throats, and fevers, while elderberry boosts the immune system and treats both sinus infections and allergies.

1¼ cup purified water

½ cup dried elderberries or 1 cup fresh (*Sambucus nigra* variety)

1 teaspoon dried mullein or 1 tablespoon fresh

1 teaspoon dried yarrow or 1 tablespoon fresh

¼ cup honey

¼ cup fresh lemon juice

If you will be using fresh herbs and berries, collect them by the waning moon or in the dawn light, when they are most saturated with water and wet with dew. If you will be using dried, mix them together, sprinkle them over a bowl containing aquamarine or turquoise, and let them sit in sunlight or near a candle for at least an hour, to soak in the healing properties of the sun.

Fill your pot with the water, then let it rest in the sun for at least ten minutes before putting it on to boil. Place clear quartz, garnet, or obsidian crystals nearby; clear quartz is a stone of generalized healing, which you can program to be more specific, while garnet invites heat and healing, specifically—good when you have a cold! Obsidian is particularly good for bacterial or viral infections. If you are sure they are completely clean and germ-free, you can place the crystals inside the water, but of course be sure to remove them before putting the pot on the stove.

Once you bring the water to a boil, simmer the berries and herbs for thirty minutes or so. Keep an eye on the water, as you don't want the pot to run dry; add more if necessary, a little at a time. Strain and allow the liquid to cool slightly. Stir in the honey and lemon juice.

Stir this syrup into hot water or tea or simply take it by the spoonful to cure a cold. It will keep in the refrigerator for a month or two.

GENTLE REST TEA

SO MANY OF US HAVE TROUBLE SLEEPING. THE PHARMA-ceutical industry—not to mention the mattress industry—profits greatly from this eternal struggle. There is so much we can do to alleviate insomnia, includ-ing exercise, meditation, and cutting back on our caffeine intake, but there are also times when it seems that no matter what we try, sleep simply will not come.

At those times, it can be helpful to get up and leave the battle for sleep behind for a little while. Spend your sleepless moments enjoying the quiet of the middle of the night—when everything is mysterious and feels ever so slightly unreal. Walk softly, and brew yourself a cup of tea that will calm your anxiety and invite rest. (Mind you, this tea will not be nearly as effective as a sleeping pill—but it likely won't cause you to sleepwalk or purchase strange items off the internet you don't remember ordering, either.)

Set a small pot of water to boil. If there's a moon out, mix your herbs in her light, using a combination of catnip, lemon balm, valerian, yarrow, and vervain. Any ratio or combination will do—each of these are peace-inducing, though valerian is particularly good for sleep. You only need a teaspoon in total for just one cup of tea. Add your herbs to a tea strainer and pour your just-boiled water over it. Allow the tea to steep for at least ten minutes, and spend this time journaling or reading. Keep the lights as dim as you can without straining your eyes. When your tea is ready, sip it slowly as you continue reading or journaling. Don't rush to finish and get back to sleep; instead, give it time to soak in. Go back to bed only when your eyes begin to feel truly heavy.

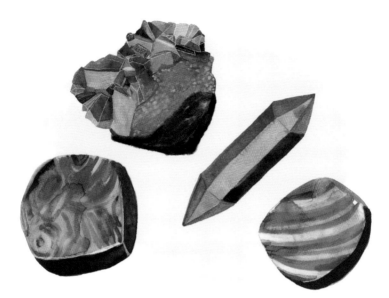

CRYSTAL LOVE RITUAL

THERE ARE SO MANY DIFFERENT KINDS OF LOVE: LOVE OF self, love of family, love of friends, romantic love, love of the earth, of Spirit, of peace and plenty. It is inarguably the most powerful force known to us and the source of all that is good and right in this world. Yet for all that, love sometimes feels so far away. It can be hard to truly sense the love given to us or the love we have to give, though both are always there. This ritual is structured to open you up to all forms of love; though if you want to focus on one in particular, you can do that as well.

You'll need only two crystals for this ritual: malachite and rose quartz. Malachite will open up your heart chakra, allowing love to flow in and out, and rose quartz will focus that love—so harness its power to place your intentions and desires for the kind of love you want to give and receive!

As with all rituals, set yourself up for greatness: Allow yourself time, and prepare a quiet, restful environment. Light some candles, and indulge in some aromatherapy by using any combination of ylang-ylang, rose, jasmine, and sandalwood essential oils in a diffuser. Set a timer for ten minutes.

Lie flat, and snuggle your shoulder blades together so that your chest is open. Place the malachite at the center of your breastbone, your heart center. Hold your rose quartz in your nondominant hand. Close your eyes.

Begin to take conscious breaths in through your nose, inhaling deeply so that you feel the malachite rise and fall, but smoothly so that it doesn't shift. As you inhale, gently squeeze the rose quartz, and open your palm up to the sky as you exhale. Allow any fears, frustrations, resentments, or sorrows to empty into your crystals—you don't have to think about those feelings and dwell on what they are. Just breathe, and allow them to go.

When your timer goes off, allow your breath to return to its normal state. Remove your stones, and sit up slowly. Take one last deep breath.

Be sure to cleanse your stones in clear water, or under the light of the moon, to remove the energy they have taken on before you use them again.

LOVE TEA

FOR SOMETHING AS POWERFUL AND NECESSARY AS LOVE, it's a good idea to employ a number of different spells and techniques to bring it forth with abundance—this is a case when more is more. This tea serves the same function as the previous crystal ritual but comes at things from a different angle, focusing less on your energies and more on your internal balance.

Because love is so very important and hard-won, there is a lot of herbal lore dedicated to manifesting it in its various forms. Some of these herbs are easier to get than others, but all of them are safe to consume in reasonable quantities:

BASIL integrates love into your daily life.

CARAWAY protects love that is already there.

CARDAMOM invites courage and passion in love.

DILL helps you sense and feel the love around you.

DITTANY is the consummate romantic love herb.

DRAGON'S BLOOD RESIN renews love that has perhaps been taken for granted.

HONEYSUCKLE invites new love.

LEMON BALM soothes love, acting as a gentle aphrodisiac.

Create your tea by choosing the herbs best suited for the qualities of love you are looking to invite into your life. You'll want a teaspoon's worth of dried herbs or a quarter cup's worth of fresh. If you're using fresh herbs, chop them roughly—just enough to release their juices and blend them together. If you're using dried herbs, grind and mix them together just a little in your mortar and pestle.

Add your herbs to your tea strainer and pour just-boiled water over them, allowing them to steep for ten minutes. Enjoy with milk and honey.

SOOTHING MEDITATION

—————

MEDITATION IS NOT EASY. WE ALL ASK OURSELVES, "AM I actually meditating now? . . . How about now?" We all chastise ourselves for thinking when instead we should be mindfully mindless. We know that this pressure we put on ourselves only makes the struggle to meditate worse, but how else can we get better? There are ways to make meditation easier. Guided meditations help us stay focused, keeping us present in the meditation. Pranayama, the art of controlling the breath, gives us something to focus on, so that the chatter of our mind can grow quiet(er). Meditative music can drown out distracting noise, both internal and external.

Each of these methods will provide a different kind of meditation for a different purpose. The aim of this meditation exercise is to soothe, to help you look for peace within yourself. Begin by rubbing lavender, chamomile, or sweet orange essential oil on the soles of your feet, where your pores are the most open. Sit *comfortably.* Use a pillow to prop up your hips and cover yourself with a blanket if you're cold—you can even lie down. Support yourself.

Take your index finger and gently close your tragus, the flap over the opening of your ear, just as if you were plugging your ears against the outside world (you are). Allow your eyes to close, but don't force them if they don't want shut. Inhale deeply through your nose. Listen to your breath. Breathe out with an audible, low-pitched hum, like a bee buzzing.

This pranayama is called Bhramari, the Humming Bee Breath, and it closes you off from all distractions, helping you find the protective space within yourself. Continue breathing in this way for as long as you like. Stop when you feel satisfied. If you want to, continue to sit in silence, reveling in that inward space you have accessed.

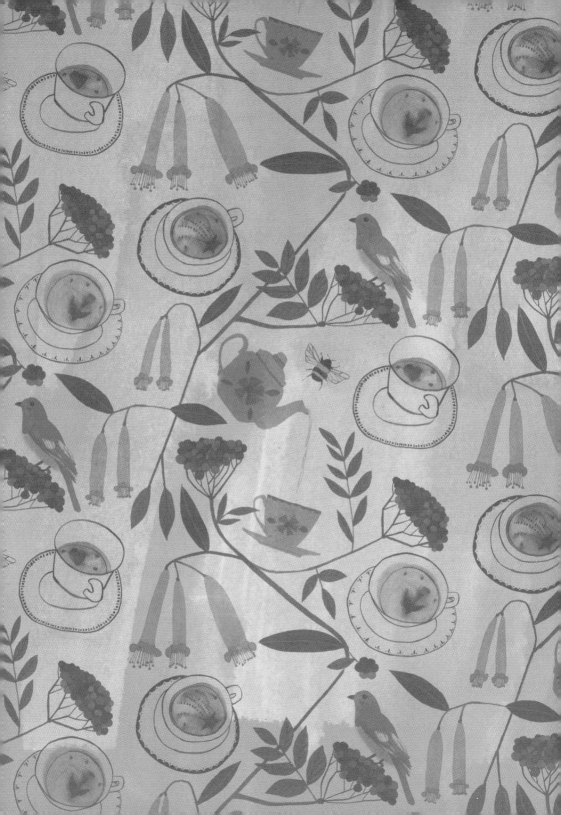

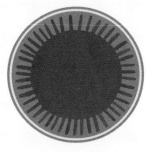

EMPOWERING

INTENTIONAL
BREAKFAST BARS

WE ALL KNOW HOW IMPORTANT BREAKFAST IS. WE ALSO ALL either skip it or eat it as quickly and absently as we can in our hurry to get on with the day. This is our reality, and there often isn't really any changing it.

These breakfast bars act as a kind of happy medium between a full sit-down meal and a gulp of coffee and a bite of bagel. They contain oregano, an adaptogenic herb that helps calm your body's response to stress, allowing you to feel clear-eyed and energetic rather than overwhelmed. They also include ginger, a natural energy enhancer; cinnamon, which improves brain function; pumpkin seeds, those veritable powerhouses of vitamins; and dried elderberries or cranberries, which increase circulation and boost the immune system. Think of them as a portable, solid potion that will energize and focus you as you face the challenges of your day.

2 cups oats

½ teaspoon salt

½ cup packed
brown sugar

½ teaspoon ground
ginger

¼ teaspoon ground
cinnamon

¼ teaspoon
oregano

½ cup dried
cranberries

½ cup pumpkin
seeds

2 tablespoons
chia seeds

¼ cup honey

6 tablespoons
melted butter

Some afternoon—*not* on a rushed morning—preheat your oven to 350 degrees, line a nine-by-nine-inch baking pan with a sheet of parchment paper, and rub some extra butter on the paper and the sides of the pan.

Begin by grinding ⅓ cup of oats in a blender or food processer until they are fine and powdery. Pour them into a large mixing bowl, and add the rest of the oats, salt, sugar, herbs, berries, and seeds. Mix them clockwise with a wooden spoon.

In a separate bowl, mix your honey with the melted butter and a tablespoon of warm water, whisking clockwise. Pour the wet ingredients into the dry ones and mix them with your hands, clumping and crumbling. Put some energy into this, as you'll get it back in the morning. Pour your mixture into the prepared baking pan, pressing it into place.

Bake for thirty to forty minutes, or until they're getting just a bit golden. They won't have set completely, and that's fine. Allow the bars to cool for about twenty minutes, then use the parchment paper to lift the baked mixture out of the pan. Place them in the refrigerator for another twenty minutes.

At this point, they will have set enough to cut into three-by-three inch bars. Store the bars in the refrigerator in an airtight container, and they will make a quick and ready breakfast—but take just a moment to savor them, to feel the energy they give before you go rushing off into your day.

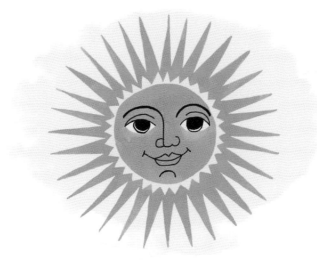

DIVINATION TEA

IT ISN'T GIVEN TO US TO KNOW THE FUTURE—NOT REALLY. And perhaps that is as it should be. This tea won't allow you to see a winning lottery number and it won't tell you whether the sun will be shining on your wedding day. What it can do is help you look inside yourself and divine what is true *for you*. It can tell you whether this new business venture you are considering is worth putting your heart into, and it can help you be certain of the love you feel for your fiancé.

This will require some work on your part. You can't just drink some tea and expect all the answers to be handed to you; you need to look deep inside yourself. This tea will help with that process and aid you in seeing your own desires and emotions clearly, but nothing and no one can do it for you.

Because we are looking inward, this tea is best consumed at night, ideally under a full moon. Set a small pot of water to boil, and mix one teaspoon's worth total of the following herbs:

LAVENDER This peaceful herb provides clarity and induces visions.

MARIGOLD Calendula is useful in prophesying, in seeing to the other side.

ROSEMARY Not only for remembrance, rosemary improves mental function and may help you understand and contextualize what you see.

WORMWOOD This extremely powerful herb should be used in small doses, and only occasionally—add it to your tea when you need an extra boost in your psychic abilities.

YARROW An herb with a long history and an even longer list of useful properties, yarrow will help enhance your perceptions.

Bruise your herbs in a mortar and pestle and then add them to your tea strainer. When your water is boiling, allow it to come to rest. When all the bubbles have subsided, pour the water over your herbs and allow them to steep for five minutes.

Sip your tea slowly. Try not to do anything else during this time—don't read, don't look at your phone, don't chat with friends and family. Sit quietly in the moonlight or other low light, and ask yourself the tough questions: What do I want? What makes me happy? What do I want to bring into the world, and what do I want to receive in return?

HOW TO READ TEA LEAVES

ALSO KNOWN AS TASSEOGRAPHY, THE ART OF READING TEA leaves dates back to the 1600s in the Western world—and perhaps earlier in other cultures. It is based on widely recognized symbolic images, including:

APPLE: Good health and good fortune.

BIRD: New information and decisions that need to be made.

BOAT: Success in a new enterprise.

BOOK: Desire for information, learning.

BROOM: Indicates a need to be sure those you are close to are good for you.

BUTTERFLY: Passing pleasure, flirtation.

CLAW: Scandal or other negative influence.

CROSS: Obstacle or other difficulty to be overcome.

CUP: Opportunity is at hand.

DRAGON: A sudden and enormous change.

EGG: New ideas, new plans.

EYE: Ability to solve difficulties, strength of character.

FEATHER: Prosperity.

HORSESHOE: Good fortune.

HOURGLASS: A warning against delay.

KEY: Indicates that your circumstances will improve.

KNIFE: A sign of strife, of broken relationships.

PALM TREE: Honor, fame, and wealth.

RABBIT: Domestic work, children.

RAVEN: Change is coming, probably negative change—or so it may seem at first.

TOADSTOOL: A warning against gossip and rash decisions.

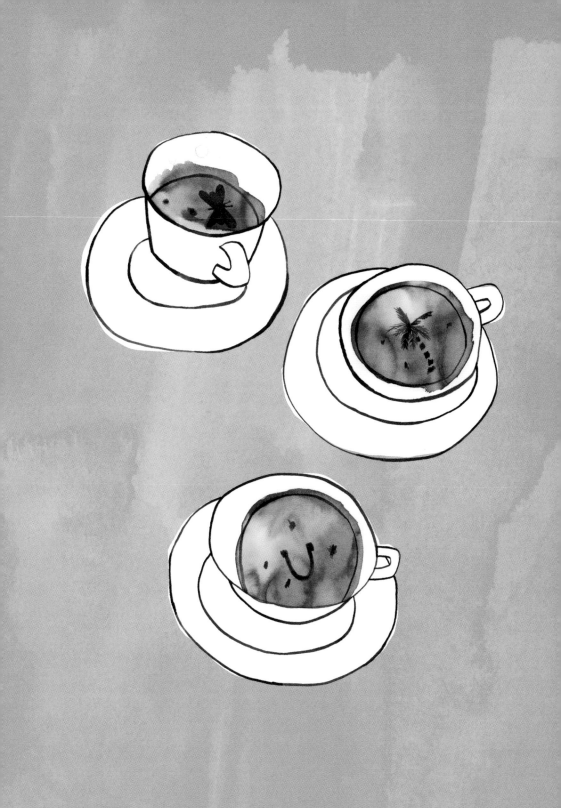

There are *lots* more symbols, but this list gives you an idea of the methodology behind tasseography: an image comes to mean something cultural (like a snake equating to betrayal), and that cultural understanding informs your reading. Now, if you are reading for yourself or someone you know well, then you might have a little more knowledge that can help inform what you see and make it more accurate (like a snake signifying your dad who loved reptiles or something like that).

To perform a reading on yourself or someone else, use a shallow white teacup with a saucer or a small plate, as this will give a greater space for the leaves to settle and allow greater visibility. Brew whatever kind of tea will best help give you the answers you seek, but add the water directly to the herbs, without using a strainer. Be sure to use small, dried herbs, as they will form clearer pictures. Allow your tea to steep for the recommended amount of time, and then drink, leaving a teaspoon or so of tea behind, along with the herbs.

Swirl the remaining tea in your cup three times. Quickly flip the teacup over and place it upside down on the saucer. Spin the cup widdershins three more times as it rests on the saucer, to dive into the mystery. Flip the cup over and peer inside. You will frequently find several images, and the meaning of one will inform the others. The handle of the cup represents the self—yourself or the person you are reading for. The rim of the cup represents the present, the sides indicate events in the near future, and the bottom of the cup is the distant future.

This is an intuitive art. At first it may feel awkward and silly, but if you trust your instincts and allow yourself to grow comfortable with the process, you will likely find it to be a useful tool in your arsenal of divination.

PSYCHIC POWER TINCTURE

GO IN UNDERSTANDING THAT THIS TINCTURE LIKELY WON'T taste all that good—but fortunately, a little of it goes a long way. Mugwort is an herb with a long history; in Norse mythology, it is one of the nine herbs of power used by the god Odin. Yarrow enhances perception and psychic abilities and was used thousands of years ago to stop bleeding on the battlefield. Anise will not only sweeten the tincture slightly, but also raise your vibrations, allowing your perceptions to soar. Mint invites clarity and positivity, to balance the power of the mugwort.

1 tablespoon dried anise or a quarter cup fresh

1 tablespoon dried mugwort or a quarter cup fresh

1 tablespoon dried yarrow or a quarter cup fresh

1 tablespoon dried mint or a quarter cup fresh

Everclear or vodka

If you are using fresh herbs, collect them by the full moon, and make the tincture that same night. If you are using dry or a combination, mix the dried herbs together and sprinkle them over a bowl that contains lapis lazuli, opal, and calcite. Charge the herbs overnight on the night just before the full moon.

On the next night, chop your fresh herbs finely, and then mix all herbs together in a mortar and pestle, breaking them down as much as possible. Place them in a jar and cover them with the Everclear or vodka. Allow the tincture to rest for one month, in darkness during the day, and in moonlight when possible.

In the light of the next full moon, strain your tincture into a dark glass container, where it will keep for months or even years. You likely will not require more than a teaspoon at a time to enhance your spellwork or meditations.

MOON MANIFESTATION RITUAL

---◦---

THE MOON SHINES MERELY WITH REFLECTED LIGHT, BUT THAT light can be so powerful it casts shadows on the ground and can be bright enough almost to read by. We know and understand that the moon, our celestial next-door neighbor, can drag the waters of oceans for miles, multiple times a day. We cannot even comprehend the effect it can have on us.

The rhythms of the moon, though mysterious, can be harnessed, as each phase of the moon's cycle brings its own power. This ritual takes you through the entire cycle, and all you need for it is a pen, paper, and a reaching mind.

the new moon

The tiniest sliver of new growth in the new moon brings with it a sense of possibility at the beginning of the waxing cycle. On this night, journal or write on individual slips of paper the things you most want to manifest in your life—be it love, creativity, abundance—anything! You can get really specific here.

the waxing moon

As the moon grows, so too do your possibilities—but unlike with the moon, these don't just happen automatically. If you want to manifest a life as a novelist, write every day, even if it's drivel. *Do your work.*

the full moon

This is your moment of power, of clarity. If you have felt for the past two weeks like you have been working in the dark, your next steps will now reveal themselves. What has been holding you back? What have you been resisting?

the waning moon

Continue to work here, but work smarter. Take the information you have been given and apply it. Don't be afraid to take a risk.

the dark moon

On this night at the end of the waning cycle, we have only the light from within to guide us. Look deep. Are you on the right journey? What has this month brought you? What have you brought to this month? Know that the cycle is about to begin again, with a new surge of possibility.

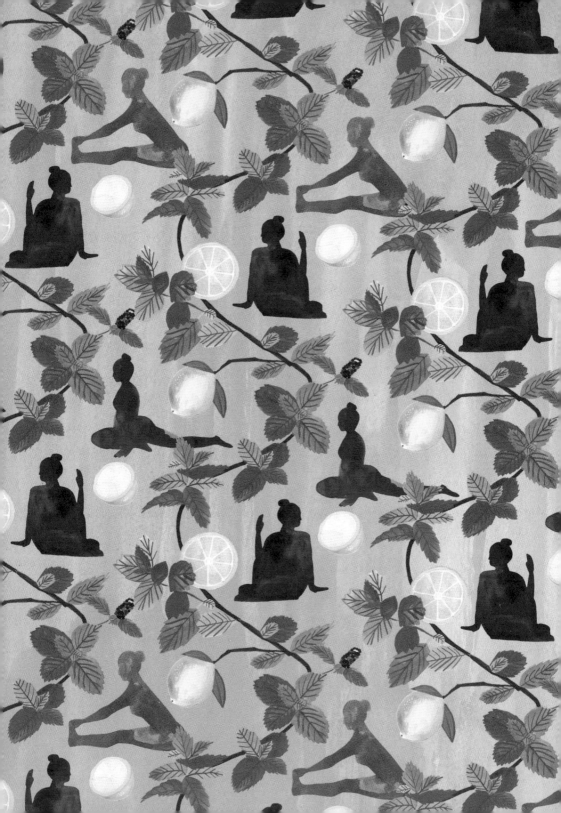

⊶ THE ⊷
EXTERNAL

We've done a lot of looking within, of tending within.
It's the most important place to begin, for all else follows
from this internal work. But it is only the beginning.

We do not live in a vacuum; we are all affected by everything
that goes on around us. A rock can scrape our knees, a harsh
word can scrape our hearts, and a thunderstorm can startle and
thrill us. We can't stop these things from happening—nor should
we—and we can't stop ourselves from being impacted by all of
this—we can only change our response to it. How can we fully
embrace a positive and find the joy or the lesson in a negative?

As always, this requires both attention and self-care.
The following rituals, balms, and intentions will help
you connect the strength within yourself to the power of
the world around you. The earth supports you.
The water blesses you. The fire ignites you.

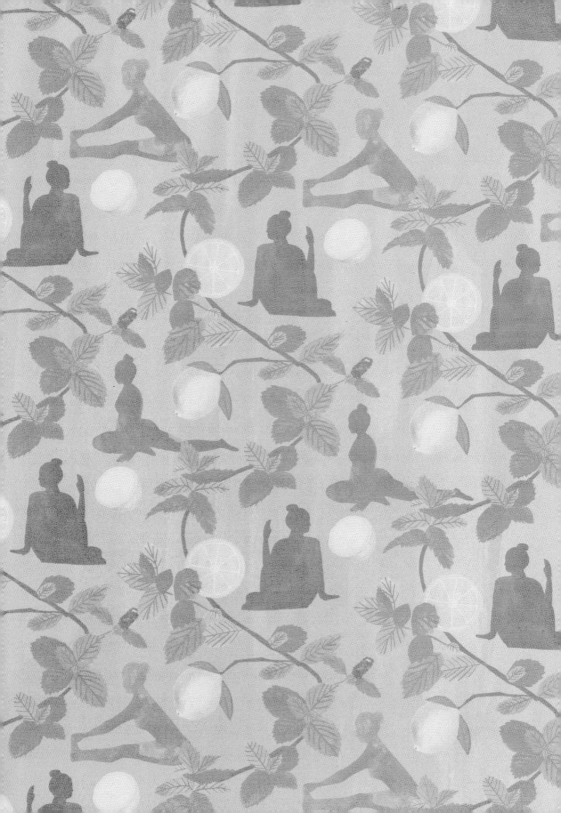

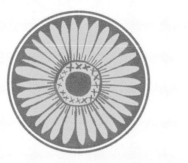

HEALING

SORE MUSCLES POULTICE

A POULTICE CAN BE ANY SORT OF SOFT, MOIST MASS USED for healing. Onion and mustard poultices were typically used as recently as the 1950s by doctors and hedge witches alike for respiratory treatments to loosen congested mucus.

That doesn't sound too terribly pleasant. But there is nothing like heat for sore muscles, and a poultice is easy to make. Arnica and comfrey are both powerful pain remedies; arnica was used by Native Americans for hundreds of years and by the Eclectic Physicians of the nineteenth and twentieth centuries, who brought botanical remedies and physical therapy into common use. Comfrey—literally known as "knitbone," is mentioned in Pliny the Elder's *Naturalis Historia* and has been used in medicine for thousands of years.

¼ cup Epsom salts

1 teaspoon arnica oil or 2 tablespoons dried arnica leaves

1 teaspoon comfrey oil or 2 tablespoons dried comfrey leaves

10–20 drops of black pepper or clove essential oil, or a combination thereof

Mix the above ingredients with enough hot water to hold them all together—adding the water a little at a time as you blend, stirring clockwise. Because you're in pain, or you're making this for someone else who is in pain and waiting for relief, there isn't a lot of time for ritual, so really put your intentions and your wishes for help and healing into your work. When it's ready, spread the poultice directly on the painful area—but only if the skin is unbroken. If you have a cut—even a small one—it's best to place a clean cotton cloth between the skin and the poultice. Allow the mixture to cool and dry, and then gently remove it with water and a clean cloth.

EUCALYPTUS HEALING OIL

EUCALYPTUS HAS A LONG TRADITION IN HEALING, PARTICULARLY in Australian Aboriginal practices. Today, it is most widely used as an aid to respiration, as it stimulates mucous membranes and clears the lungs. Juniper's reputation for protection, purification, and healing enhances the power of the eucalyptus, and both bring the growth, power, and reliability of their trees. Depending on when you want to use this unguent, adding lime peel invites brightness and vitamin C. If you're planning to apply this oil just before going to sleep, skip the citrus.

4 ounces eucalyptus leaves, fresh or dried

1 ounce juniper berries, fresh or dried

2 ounces lime peel, fresh (optional)

Olive or almond oil (carrier)

If you are using fresh eucalyptus leaves and juniper berries, collect them early to midmorning on a bright clear day. Chop them finely, and the lime peel as well if you will be using this. If you will be working with dried leaves and berries, sprinkle them over a bowl containing turquoise and clear quartz. Allow them to sit in the sunshine for an hour.

Mix all your ingredients except the oil in your mortar and pestle, bruising and integrating them. Place the resulting paste in a small jar and cover it with your carrier oil. Allow the mixture to rest in sunlight for six weeks, then apply to the chest or beneath the nose to ease respiration and clear the head.

AYURVEDIC MASSAGE OIL

ONE OF THE MANY TRADITIONS OF AYURVEDA IS REGULAR massage, also known as Bahya Snehana. It's basically a form of lubrication for the body, to keep everything moving smoothly and painlessly. Sesame oil is traditionally used in Ayurvedic medicine, but you can try another oil like sweet almond or avocado oil if you prefer. Ginger will stimulate your muscles, encouraging circulation. Turmeric, a natural anti-inflammatory, improves joint function, and cardamom reduces swelling, while inviting a sense of comfort and well-being.

---

3 ounces sesame oil

10 drops ginger essential oil

10 drops turmeric essential oil

10 drops cardamom essential oil

Mix all the ingredients well, and store this oil in a dark glass jar or bottle, allowing at least a week in a dark space, surrounded by yellow jasper, pyrite, jade, and citrine, before use. When the oil is ready, massage it into your feet, onto your scalp, or over your entire body, focusing on your joints. Follow the massage by adding heat to your body—either by sitting in the sun, performing a gentle yoga practice, or taking a bath. If you can, rest for the remainder of the day, allowing the benefits to seep in.

INTERNAL MASSAGE YOGA PRACTICE

SOMETIMES, YOU HAVE TO GET A LITTLE FARTHER THAN JUST skin-deep. There is a flow of energy within us—it's known as *prana* in yoga, but you may have heard it referred to as *qi* or energy meridians or *nadis*. Our *prana* is our life force, and we are at our best when it is flowing smoothly through us—and even out beyond us into the world. That smooth current of energy requires tending, from time to time, as we become blocked by frustration, by toxins in the air and in the foods we eat, by stress, by emotion—by all the things we experience as we make our way through life. These five yoga poses can be done in a gentle sequence, or asana, and together they will wring out your system, detoxing and loosening up that flow of energy.

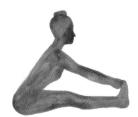

paschimottanasana
(SEATED FORWARD FOLD)

Begin by sitting on the floor with your legs extended in front of you, pointing your toes to the sky, keeping the legs hip-width apart. Align your spine as straight as possible. Then dig your heels into the ground and bend your knees slightly. Raise your arms straight up overhead and reach them forward past your feet, grabbing onto your outer arches if you can. Take a deep breath in, and as you exhale, lower your forehead to your knees. If it feels comfortable to do so, straighten your legs. Stay here for three breaths.

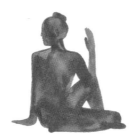

ardha matsyendrasana
(SEATED SPINAL TWIST)

Extend both legs out again in a seated position, with your spine straight. Lift your right leg and cross it over the left, bringing your right foot to the floor over by your left thigh and your right knee pointing up to the sky. Fold the left leg at the knee, with toes pointing behind you. Hook your left elbow around your right knee and extend your right hand to the floor behind your right hip to support you. Use your left elbow to help shift your torso to the right, looking over your right shoulder and opening your heart wide. Be gentle with yourself. Stay here for three breaths, then unwind your limbs and repeat on the other side.

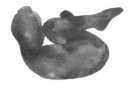

pavanamuktasana
(WIND-RELIEVING POSE)

Scooch your hips forward and lower yourself onto your back, bringing your knees up to your chest. Wrap your arms around your knees and gently lift your head and chest so that your nose brushes your knees—or that's the intention anyway, listen to your body as you find what works for you. Stay here for three breaths.

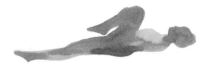

supta matsyendrasana
(RECLINED SPINAL TWIST)

Lower your head and chest, and extend your right leg out long, keeping your left leg tucked into your chest. Use your right arm to bring your left knee over to the right side of your body, intending to keep your right shoulder on the ground while your left knee approaches it. Turn your head to look past your left shoulder. Stay here for three breaths, then unwind your limbs and repeat on the other side.

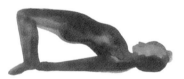

setu bandha sarvangasana
(BRIDGE POSE)

Bring your knees together, so that they are facing the sky, with both feet on the ground. Place your feet hip-width apart, and just a little farther from your seat than your extended arms can reach. Place your palms flat on the ground and inhale. As you exhale, lift your hips to the sky, keeping your feet and palms flat. Inhale, and exhale to release back to the ground. Repeat this sequence twice more.

GENTLE SHAMPOO
+ CONDITIONER

THE WELLNESS WITCH IS A THRIFTY GAL AND OFTEN APPALLED at how much money we spend on our hair—and by the damage we do to Mother Earth with chemicals. Our relationship with the earth is the source of our power, and we honor it by living as naturally as we can.

Making your own shampoo is so much easier than it seems, particularly because it mostly relies upon an inexpensive, gentle soap that is readily available for purchase: liquid castile soap. Castile soap is a cleanser made with a vegetable-based oil, rather than an animal fat (originally just olive oil, it now includes anything from coconut oil to hempseed oil to . . . whatever other plant readily produces oil). The most popular brand is Dr. Bronner's, but there are others.

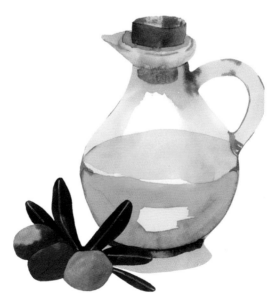

shampoo

Your shampoo will be thinner and runnier than you might be used to and won't be nearly as sudsy, but it is a gentler, more environmentally friendly approach to healthy hair. If you want to thicken and emulsify your products, you can add something called BTMS, an emulsifier developed from rapeseed oil.

FOR DRY HAIR USE:

Chamomile

Aloe

Calendula/marigold

Peppermint

FOR OILY HAIR USE:

Rosemary

Lemongrass

Ginger

Lemon peel

1 cup of castile soap

2 tablespoons vegetable glycerin

2 teaspoons argan oil

80 drops of essential oil, using a blend that aligns with your herbal choices

1 tablespoon aloe vera gel (optional)

First, determine your hair needs: Is your hair usually dry or does it tend to be oily? If you have a combination of these (e.g., oily at the scalp but dry down at the ends), err on the side of how your roots behave.

Do you shower in the morning or at night? If you shower at night, begin your work in the evening, and if you shower in the morning, start in the morning. Collect ¼ cup of your appropriate herbs, fresh or dried. Use fresh aloe if you have it, but if you have to resort to aloe vera gel, hold off on adding it until later in the process. Bring one cup of water to a boil, and then pour it over your herbs. Allow the herbs to steep in the liquid overnight surrounded by moonstone, amethyst, and rose quartz, or throughout the day, incorporating sunstone, aquamarine, and pyrite.

Strain the water, and pour it into a mixing bowl. Add the rest of the ingredients. Mix well, pour into an empty shampoo bottle, and use freely, without worrying about overdrying your hair.

conditioner

This process is remarkably similar to making shampoo. Brew your herbal water using the same ingredients and the same method. Add it to a spray bottle, along with two tablespoons of filtered apple cider vinegar (*not* the raw kind—that would clog the sprayer) and around forty drops of your essential oil blend. The vinegar will balance the pH of your hair, reducing frizz, and actually detangle it as well. After shampooing, spray the conditioner onto your hair and let it sit for a few minutes before rinsing; don't worry, the vinegar scent won't last once your hair is dry.

Every once in a while (once a month if you have oily hair, twice a month if your hair is dry), give yourself a hair oil treatment.

FOR DRY HAIR USE:

> 2 tablespoons coconut oil
>
> 2 tablespoons argan oil
>
> 5 drops essential oils of your chosen blend

FOR OILY HAIR USE:

> 2 tablespoons coconut oil
>
> 2 tablespoons jojoba oil
>
> 5 drops essential oils of your chosen blend

Heat the coconut oil in a microwave just until it reaches a liquid state, and stir in your other ingredients. Work the oil into your hair, paying special attention to the ends, and leave it in for half an hour. Sit in the sun if you can, allowing its warmth to help the oils penetrate.

Oily hair is often caused by an imbalance in pH—the jojoba oil we are using here is your best bet for nourishing your ends while not causing your roots to feel like an oil slick.

EARTHING RITUAL

FROM TIME TO TIME, AND MORE AND MORE OFTEN THESE DAYS, we all need to take a moment to ground ourselves, to regain our inner peace, to connect with the earth and be healed by the land, returning our energies to it and healing the earth in turn. Nothing is needed for this ritual but time and intention, although certain items can assist your practice:

○ Hematite crystal, a stone of protection and grounding, will seal out negative forces. Alternatively, you could program clear quartz to serve the same purpose.

○ A smudge wand, perhaps with sage, lavender, and thyme

○ An essential oil blend featuring any of the above

○ Access to the earth, either grass or dirt. If this is not feasible, get as low to the floor as you can.

Cleanse your space with a smudge wand if you like, and dab a little essential oil on your temples and the soles of your feet. Sit comfortably on the ground. Hold your crystal lightly in your palm, or sit with your hands in your lap.

Close your eyes and allow awareness of your surroundings to capture your attention. Feel the air on your face, the touch of the floor or grass or earth beneath you, and the smells and sounds surrounding you. Continue to breathe slowly and deeply, making your inhalations and exhalations the same length, and smoothing out the pause in between.

Feel your connection to that which is beneath you. Allow your breath to sync with the natural pulse, the ebb and flow of the earth. Let your mind drift, and continue to breathe.

When you feel ready, allow your eyes to open slowly and gently. Take a final deep breath, and bow your head to your chest. When you rise to your feet, do so with intention, feeling the earth beneath you and supporting you.

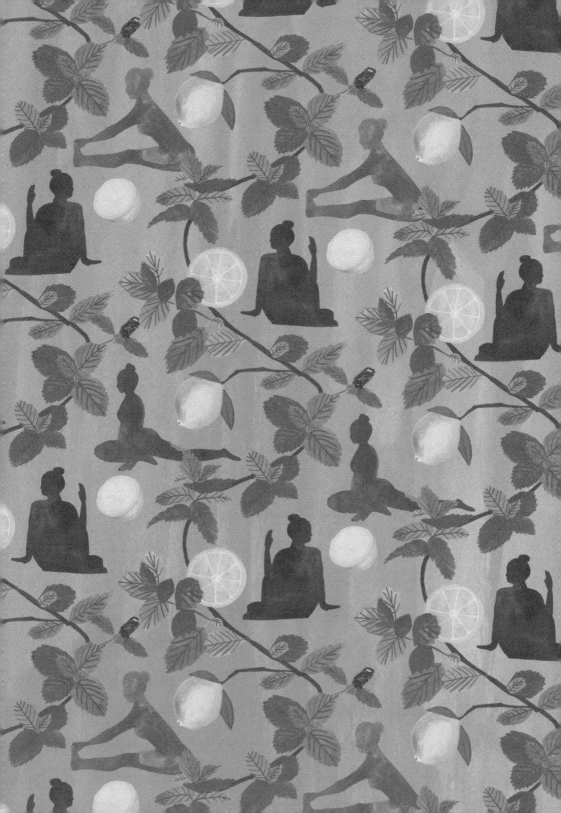

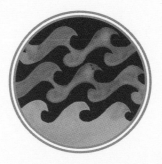

SOOTHING

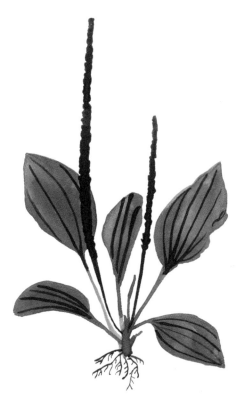

PLANTAIN AND HONEY BRUISE AND STING SALVE

PLANTAIN—THE HERB, NOT THE BANANA—IS A WEED. IT GROWS, undeterred, in just about every lawn in America, and we're always trying to get it out. But the thing is, it's actually an extremely beneficial herb, as it acts as an antimicrobial and anti-inflammatory analgesic, *and* it helps with tissue regeneration. Honey is another antibacterial substance. Together they can soothe and protect your skin from cuts, scrapes, stings, and bites.

Gather enough plantain leaves to fill a small jar. Wash and dry them, and then roughly tear or chop them, just to release their juices. Cover them with an inch or so of the oil of your choice—coconut oil or olive oil are excellent options for skin care and relief from minor aches and abrasions. Close the jar and leave it in the sun for at least six weeks. Surround the jar with citrine, garnet, obsidian, pyrite, and turquoise. Then follow this recipe to make the final salve. Then follow this recipe to make the final salve.

¼ cup herbal oil

¼–½ ounce beeswax

1 tablespoon honey

30 drops of a combination of chamomile, helichrysum, lavender, or patchouli essential oils

Strain your ¼ cup of herbal oil into a small saucepan and heat it at a low temperature. Add the ¼–½ ounce of beeswax, depending on how soft or firm you want your salve to be. When the beeswax has melted, add the honey and the essential oils, and pour this mixture back into your jar to cool. Spread your salve directly onto stings, bites, bruises, and small cuts. Once you've done so, cup your palm over the injury, allowing your heat, energy, and healing intention to penetrate.

RELAXING BATH SALTS

BATH SALTS ARE SHOCKINGLY EASY TO MAKE AND UTILIZE ingredients that you likely already have in your cupboard. The surprising thing is that arguably the best kind of salt for your body—Epsom salts—is not actually a "salt" at all. It's a naturally occurring mineral compound of magnesium and sulfate and provides all sorts of benefits from reducing inflammation to improving muscle function to flushing toxins, while helping the body absorb nutrients. Baking soda, another natural mineral compound, also helps flush toxins, while at the same time healing and soothing the skin.

1 cup Epsom salts

1 cup baking soda

½ cup dried herbs (including roses, calendula, or lavender)

Food coloring (optional)

20–30 drops of an essential oil blend of your choice (lavender, rose, or peppermint are good options)

Mason jar

Blend your Epsom salts and baking soda in a bowl. Mix in your dried herbs. Add a few drops of food coloring if you like, as well as your essential oils, and mix it all together. Stir widdershins to invoke rest, and as you do so, visualize the images that most inspire relaxation in you—whether that's lying in a hammock, sunbathing, or swimming amongst the stars. Store in the mason jar.

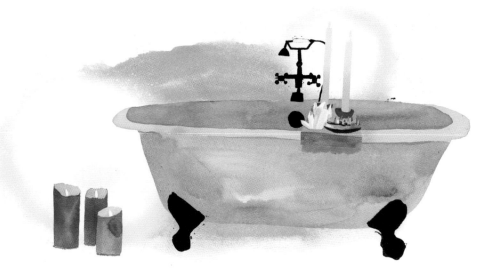

HEALING BATH RITUAL

FROM OUR INFANCY, WE HAVE TAKEN COMFORT AND HEALING in the power of baths. Cultures around the world from Iceland to Russia to Japan view bathing as a ritual—a practice that is done with intention and reflection. You don't need a giant claw-foot bathtub, much less a hot spring, to enjoy a healing soak; as long as you can immerse yourself in enough water to relax, you've got everything you need.

Of course, it's always nice to add a little extra! Consider gathering these materials and preparing the following experience, to make this ritual even more curative.

1 cup Relaxing Bath Salts (see page 72)

1 sprig each of fresh vervain, rue, lemon balm, or lavender

Candles

A glass of water

Soothing music

Start by alerting anyone in your household that you will need at least one hour of undisturbed time. Turn off all notifications from your phone. Select your music, playing it at a low enough volume to allow you to drift off, but loud enough to mostly drown out the noise of the world around you. Clean all extraneous items out of your bathtub—you want a clear space. Set your lighting, get your beverage ready, and begin to draw your bath.

Make it as hot or cool as you like, depending on the season and your body's needs. As the water flows, add your salts and your herbs. Before you get in, lean over the tub, stirring it counterclockwise. As you stir, set your intention for this bath. How will you feel during the ritual? How will you feel afterward? If you can, speak these intentions aloud, as the water will retain and be altered by the vibrations of your voice. When you are ready, step into the tub.

And then—just be. Sip your water. Splash. Close your eyes. Let the soothing music wash over you. Spend as much or as little time in the bath as you want. Allow your body and mind to relax, and ask as little of yourself as you can.

When you feel ready, step out. If it's warm enough or practical to air-dry, do so—but don't rinse off. Allow the tub to drain, and fish out any petals or herbs floating in the water. Allow them to dry a bit, and if it's practical to do so, either bury them or add them to a compost pile. Return them, and their energy, to the earth.

SWEET DREAMS BALM

THOSE OF US WHO OPEN OUR MINDS TO THAT WHICH IS beyond our ordinary consciousness can occasionally find that unwelcome visions, thoughts, or energies make their way through our doors—often in the form of nightmares. Nightmares, of course, serve a crucial function, as our subconscious works out all that might be troubling us. On the other hand, a restful sleep is the most important thing we can do for ourselves, so if you find that nightmares are too frequent a visitor, this balm will ease your dreams.

¼ cup herbal oil

¼ ounce beeswax, grated

15 drops lavender essential oil

10 drops sweet orange essential oil

Create an herbal oil, as on page 59, with a scent you find soothing and peaceful. Collect sweetgrass, use a vanilla bean, or incorporate any other scent that reminds you of safety, sweetness, and gentleness. If you have one already made, use that, or create one by covering your chosen ingredient with an unscented carrier oil like expeller-pressed grapeseed oil, and let it sit in sunlight for six weeks, surrounded by amethyst, lapis lazuli, moonstone, and rose quartz.

Heat a quarter cup of the oil over very low heat just until you can feel the warmth rising. Add the beeswax and stir clockwise until it has melted. Remove from the heat and pour the mixture in a mason jar. Add your essential oils and stir. Cover and let it set for two hours. Rub it gently on your chest and the soles of your feet as you climb into bed.

YIN YOGA PRACTICE

ESSENTIALLY, YIN YOGA IS THE PRACTICE OF HOLDING POSES
for a longer period of time, rather than flowing through them in an asana. This
technique can help build strength and ease in the body without placing undue
stress on it. Although advanced practitioners hold difficult poses like Side Crow
for several minutes, the series of poses we will work with allows your body to
relax into the stretch, letting gravity do the work, rather than fighting it for an
extended period of time. It will help your body release the tension and emotion
it carries for you and elevate your meditation practice, as your body becomes
more used to being still.

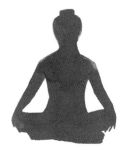

sukhasana
(CROSS-LEGGED POSE)

Translating to the "pose of ease," Sukhasana brings back elementary school
memories of sitting on the classroom carpet—and yet, it's not particularly
easy or comfortable. Bring a folded towel or a pillow under your hips, allowing
your pelvis to tilt forward, so that your knees are below your hip socket. Sit
as straight as you can, trying to keep your heart aligned over your hips, and
your head aligned over your heart. Imagine your seven chakras—your root, your
sacral chakra, your solar plexus, your heart, your throat, your third eye, and your
crown—all connecting in a straight line that stretches from the earth up to the

heavens. Engage your core slightly, as this will help you sit up straight without placing undue strain on your back. Place your palms on your knees, hands open so that you can receive whatever is being offered, and lift your chest to the sky with each breath in. Stay here for at least two minutes.

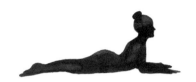

salamba bhujangasana
(SPHINX POSE)

Beginning facedown, place your elbows directly under your shoulders, with your palms flat on the earth at a ninety-degree angle with your biceps. Claw into your fingertips, allowing your arms to take your weight, as your lower back softens. Tuck your chin slightly so you don't stress your neck. Feel yourself rise slightly as you breathe deeply, staying for at least two minutes.

utthita balasana
(EXTENDED CHILD'S POSE)

From a kneeling position, bring your toes together and spread your knees so that they are wider than your hips. Extend your arms forward and lower your body to the earth, bringing your forehead to the ground if you can. Keep your arms outstretched and your palms flat, allowing your hips to sink back onto your feet. Feel your back stretch as you breathe, remaining still for at least two minutes.

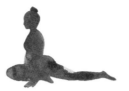

eka pada rajakapotasana
(PIGEON POSE)

Starting from all fours, bring your right knee up toward your right wrist, and move your right foot out toward your left—if you're superflexible and careful with your knee, you can work to bring your right foot as far forward as you can, but start by keeping it close to your body. Extend your left leg out straight behind you, and slowly relax your torso over your bent right knee, lowering onto your forearms or even your forehead, if your body allows it. Breathe deeply, feeling your belly against your right leg, for at least two minutes, and then switch to the other side.

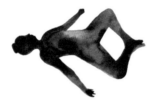

supta baddha konasana
(RECLINED BOUND ANGLE)

Lie flat on your back and draw the soles of your feet together, with your knees extending out to the sides. Place your hands palms down, arms extending out from your sides. Breathe deeply, feeling your belly rise between and above your hands. Don't push your legs down to the earth, but allow them to fall as they release. Stay here for at least two minutes.

WATER RITUAL

JUST ABOUT EVERY CULTURE IN THE WORLD FINDS MAGIC in water. This seems obvious, because, of course, we rely on water to stay alive—and yet, no more so than with any other element. But water's qualities of purification, as well as its sense of protection, even forgiveness, which is nevertheless shrouded in mystery, make it eternally, subtly powerful. It holds us up, it washes us clean, it sustains us, and it is the very essence of renewal.

To immerse yourself in those qualities, wait for a rainy day. If you can, hold out for a really drenching rain, not just a light drizzle. Keeping the rest of your body dry, extend your palms out beneath the sky, so you can feel the individual drops of water as they slap and break on your skin. Bow your head and step out into the rain. Let it fall on your head and shoulders, massaging you, until water begins to drip down your face. Slowly, with your eyes closed, raise your face to the sky.

Look inside. What is the rain asking of you? If it is bringing forth tears, let them fall to mingle with the raindrops. Do you want to run back inside and curl up under a blanket with a cup of tea? Or do you want to go find some puddles to stomp in? Let the rain renew you.

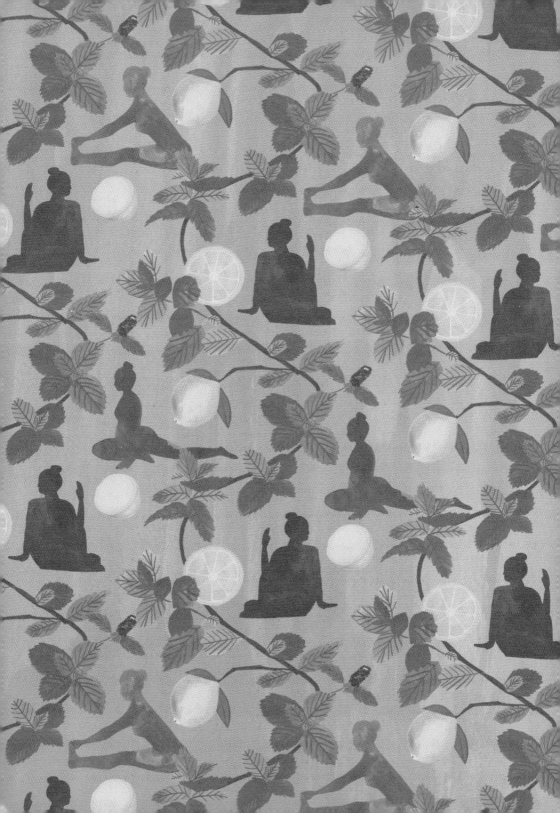

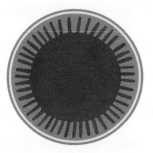

EMPOWERING

FINDING YOUR VOICE LIP BALM

THE THROAT CHAKRA IS THE MOST EASILY BLOCKED OF OUR power centers. We can feel completely unable to speak our truths or to live our own lives with joy and pride. This lip balm will activate your throat chakra and bring forth your authentic voice.

Or, you know, you could just add it to your eternal lip balm collection—because you can *never* have too many.

1–2 teaspoons beeswax

2 teaspoons coconut oil

2 teaspoons shea butter

Small jar or tin

Over very low heat, melt the beeswax, coconut oil, and shea butter in a saucepan. You will want more beeswax if you live in a warmer environment, and less if your house stays cool. Gently stir clockwise until the oils are well-blended. Remove the pan from the heat. Carefully pour the mixture into your small jar. As you allow it to cool, surround it with turquoise or aquamarine stones, so they can infuse your lip balm with their strength.

RISE AND SHINE TONER

TONER GOES IN AND OUT OF FASHION AS A BEAUTY PRODUCT, but its efficacy as a wake-up call to the mind and spirit is without question. A bright spritz on sleepy, closed eyes can clear your head, invite new energy, and invigorate you to move forward into your day with a lightness of spirit. And if it clarifies the skin, too? Well, that's just a bonus.

Witch hazel, the plant with just about the most magical name ever, is a botanical that contains tannins (the same compounds found in red wine) capable of reducing skin inflammation, preventing acne, and fighting bacteria. All-natural, alcohol-free brands of witch hazel extract will tone your skin without drying it, as an astringent would. Vitamin C is also excellent for your skin, as it helps you maintain a slightly acidic pH (which fends off bacteria and fungi) while at the same time working to combat free radicals. Please note, though, that vitamin C can make your skin more light-sensitive, so be sure to apply a sunscreen when heading outdoors.

---

3 ounces water

1 grapefruit

3 ounces alcohol-free witch hazel extract

10–20 drops tea tree oil to assist in fighting bacteria

10–20 drops chamomile oil to soothe the skin

glass spray bottle

Bring the water to a boil. As it is heating, wash the grapefruit well and then peel the outer zest off with a vegetable peeler. Pour the boiled water over the grapefruit peel and allow this to steep until it has reached room temperature.

Strain out the grapefruit, and stir the witch hazel extract and essential oils into the infused water. Store the spritz in a glass spray bottle.

THE FIVE RITES

THE SERIES OF MOVEMENTS KNOWN AS THE FIVE RITES IS A practice said to be rooted in Tibet and dating back 2,500 years. This is a much more vigorous effort than the restorative yoga poses we've explored so far (see page 61 and 76), but the benefits are worth it: regular practice increases strength, energy, and flexibility and reduces stress, while inviting a deeper clarity of thought and a greater sense of personal power.

Between each rite, stand up straight and take two deep, cleansing breaths.

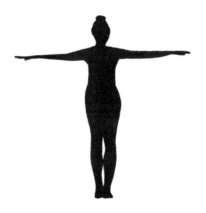

the first rite

While standing, stretch out your arms into a T-shape. Spin around, with your arms out like a helicopter, as fast as you can until you become dizzy. Welcome the child-at-play energy into your body.

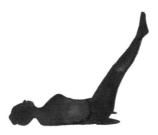

the second rite

Lie down flat on the ground, placing your hands palm down next to your hips. Raise your legs up into the air, toes to the ceiling, legs as straight as you can make them, allowing your head, neck, and shoulders to follow them up, being careful to avoid crunching the neck. You're resting on your lower back. Stay there for a breath, then slowly lower your upper back, legs, and feet to the floor. Stay there for a breath, allowing your body to relax completely. Repeat this motion five times.

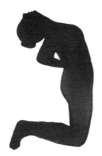

the third rite

Kneel with your toes curled under for stability. Placing your palms against your thighs, curve your upper spine, angling your nose toward your navel. Stay there for a breath. Rise back up and arch your upper spine, angling your nose to the ceiling. Stay there for a breath, and repeat this sequence five times.

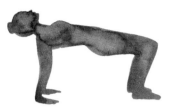

the fourth rite

Sit on the earth with your legs straight out in front of you, toes to the sky and palms flat on the earth beside you. Lower your chin to your chest. Stay there for a breath, then bend your knees as you pull your hips up toward the sky, keeping your arms straight and dropping your head back toward the earth. Stay here for a breath, and repeat this sequence five times.

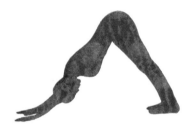

the fifth rite

Essentially, this rite involves moving back and forth from Adho Mukha Svanasana (Downward-Facing Dog) to Urdhva Mukha Svanasana (Upward-Facing Dog). Begin with your hands on the ground and your hips shooting up in the air, legs and arms straight with weight evenly distributed between your two hands and two feet. Take a deep breath. Then lower your hips, pulling your upper body between your arms, and arching your chest up to the sky as your feet curl so that their tops and your hands are the only parts of your body that touch the ground. Take another deep breath, and repeat this sequence five times.

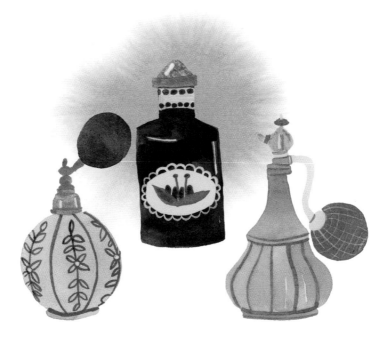

COURAGEOUS PERFUME OIL

FIRST OF ALL, LET'S NOTE THAT PERFUME OIL IS *STRONG*, much stronger than your average over-the-counter eau de cologne, as it can contain as much as 80 percent fragrance oils (the rest being an unscented carrier oil). It can, of course, be less fragrant, should you want a lighter scent, but this is *courageous* perfume oil, intended to spur you on an adventure. Strength is a must.

All good perfumes contain three notes, like a chord on a piano: a base note, a middle note, and a top note. The base note is long-lasting and shows a lot of depth, the middle note is a bit like a horse at the head of the pack in a race—it comes out first and hard. The top note is generally more fleeting—it's the scent that disappears as your perfume settles into your skin, leaving a lingering memory.

All perfumes smell differently on different people, as we all have our own individual scents and body chemistry. So you will need to tinker with this recipe, much like you would a spell or potion, and figure out what works best for you! Here are a variety of essential oils, each of which will enhance your power and vitality.

BASE NOTES	MIDDLE NOTES	TOP NOTES
Black spruce	Ginger	Frankincense
Cedarwood	Juniper	Lemon
Myrrh	Neroli	Lime
Opopanax	Palo santo	Sweet orange
Clove	Tea tree oil	Peppermint
Cinnamon	Thyme	Piñon
		Rosemary

Because your base note needs to carry your perfume through, you'll want to create a mixture of two parts base note, one part middle note, and one part top note. So, for instance, you could combine twenty drops of cedarwood, ten drops of neroli, and ten drops of frankincense. Add one teaspoon sweet almond, grapeseed, or another unscented carrier oil, and store this perfume oil in a small dark glass bottle. When using your perfume, set your intention for courage as you apply it to your inner wrists and temples.

LOVE AND BE LOVED BODY CREAM

CHOCOLATE IS KNOWN THE WORLD OVER AS A SYMBOL OF love and sensuality. The main ingredient in this cream is cocoa butter, which retains a bit of chocolate's distinctive scent, along with its loving and healing properties. Cardamom, clove, cinnamon, ginger, caraway, and rose—these and many other herbs have been used for centuries to invite and enhance love, both for ourselves and those around us. Obviously, they shouldn't all be used at once—certain combinations work better for certain people. You should adjust the scents according to what works for your sense of self, your body chemistry, and your energy. Consider what sort of love you are looking to enhance in your life.

¼ cup coconut oil

½ cup cocoa butter

¼ cup avocado oil

30 drops total of your chosen essential oil blend

Melt the coconut oil and cocoa butter over very low heat. Stir until just blended, either clockwise or counterclockwise, depending on whether you're inviting friendly, familial love, or a more sensual, romantic love. Remove your pot from the heat. Pour the mixture into a wide-mouthed jar and stir in your essential oils. Refrigerate the jar for three to four hours or until the mixture has started to thicken.

Using a stand or hand mixer, whip the mixture on high for ten minutes. Pour it back into your wide-mouthed jar and refrigerate for another three to four hours. Should the temperature in your home rise over seventy-five degrees, you may need to chill and rewhip.

You can use this cream every day to soothe dry skin; it will both invite and give love.

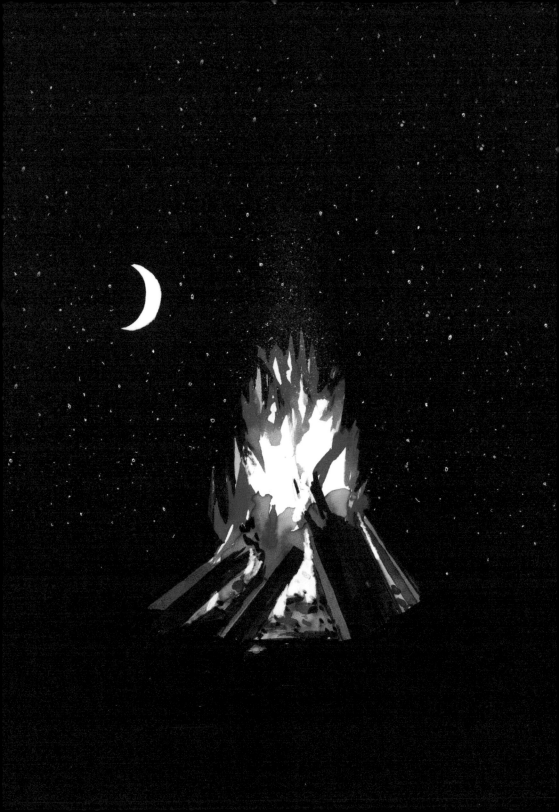

FIRE RITUAL

FIRE. IT IS WHAT LIGHTS US, WHAT DESTROYS US, AND WHAT spurs us ever onward. It is motion, it is danger, it is power made manifest.

We can harness this power and use it to our advantage. There's no need to walk through it or anything—but symbolically we can call on the nature of fire to destroy anything that has been holding us back.

This can be done with a candle, a campfire, or even a roaring bonfire, depending on how much force you require—so ask yourself, what are you going to burn? Is it an object, like a shirt you wore on a traumatic day? Or is it a piece of paper with your worst fears scribbled on it? That will determine the kind of fire you need.

Whether you're conjuring with a crackling campfire or a flickering tea light, be safe! If you're working with a candle, make sure it's on a stable surface with a plate underneath to catch any ash, and check there isn't a draft from an open window. If you're working with an outdoor fire, make sure you're not in a drought and that you have adequate protections and fire extinguishers nearby, just in case.

Once your fire is lit and ready, hold the object in your hand. Really look at it. This is the last time you're going to see it, so take a moment to confront that fact. When you put your object into the fire, do so with intention. Say goodbye. Your goodbye can be with gratitude for the knowledge your fears have given you, with venom for the damage they have done, or with an utter dismissal of something that no longer matters. Know and understand in yourself what kind of ending this is.

Watch it burn. This may take no time at all, or it may take several minutes. Be there for the whole process. When there is nothing left of your object but ash, douse the flame and walk away. You're done with it.

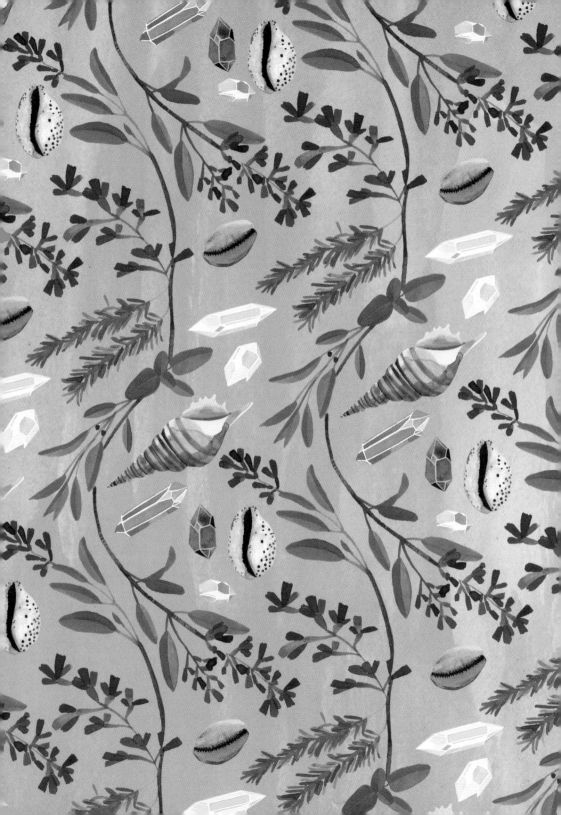

⟶ THE ⟵
HOME

*We are profoundly influenced by our surroundings,
and if we can make of our home a haven,
one that is both a sanctuary and a power center,
we can enhance our gifts and our potential tenfold.*

*The home is the hearth and heart of any
wellness witch's practice. It is both the source
and the outcome of all that we do.
The practices, spells, and curios offered here
will help to transform your home—the place
you return to and leave from every day—into the
setting that will protect you, recharge you,
and purify you.*

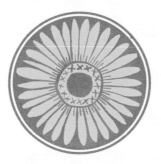

HEALING

CLEANING SPRAY

}—o—{

IT IS BEST TO START FRESH, IN BOTH MAGIC AND LIFE. THIS all-natural and very effective cleaning spray will boot out the old and make room for the new, leaving your home smelling airy and bright, without introducing the energy of harsh chemicals.

1 cup distilled white vinegar

4 strips of lemon peel

2 cups water

20 drops tea tree essential oil

20 drops lemon essential oil

20 drops peppermint essential oil

Dark glass spray bottle

Heat the vinegar until it just simmers, then add the lemon peel. Allow it to simmer for ten minutes, then remove the lemon peel and let the vinegar to cool to room temperature, surrounded by turquoise, obsidian, and clear quartz. Stir in the remaining ingredients and pour the mixture into your spray bottle.

WHITE SANDALWOOD CANDLE

CANDLES HAVE BEEN A PART OF RELIGIOUS AND SPIRITUAL practices for centuries, as they literally *bring light*. These days, barring a power outage, we don't use candles for their original purpose; instead, we look to them as a kind of invocation. Candles can bring sensuality, peacefulness, meditativeness, a sense of occasion, and so much more.

Here, we are inviting peace. The color white represents safety, purity, and cleanliness. It is the absence of color, allowing us to be without influence. We add to that by scenting our candle with sandalwood, a sweet, woody fragrance that can clear out energies, leaving behind only a gentle, meditative uplift.

Double boiler
(It's probably best to use one specifically for candlemaking, as cleaning out the wax is a pain.)

½ pound soy wax

Wick

8 ounce jar

Sandalwood fragrance oil
(not essential oil, which doesn't last)

Wick holder

Using your double boiler, melt your wax slowly. As the wax melts, dip the bottom of your wick into the liquid, and use this to affix the wick in the center of your jar, holding it in place until the wax hardens (this will only take a few moments).

When your wax has turned entirely liquid, remove it from the heat and stir in up to half an ounce of your fragrance oil, blending it well. Run your jar under hot water to warm it up a bit. Dry it well, and then pour the wax carefully into this vessel. Use the wick holder to keep the wick upright and let the candle cool for thirty to sixty minutes before you remove it.

HEALING SIGIL

SIGIL MAGIC HAS ITS ROOTS IN WHAT APPEARS, AT FIRST glance, to be fairly dark history: a pentagram is a sigil. Of course, a pentagram was never intended to be some kind of demon-summoning spell—it was and still is a symbol of protection—but the connotation of darker forces is there.

The reality of sigil magic is much brighter—in fact, it's artistic, creative, and really *fun*. A sigil is created by writing out an intention, then scrambling that intention so that it is unrecognizable, even to the caster, thus allowing the spell to go forth and do its work without conscious influence from the witch herself.

Start with something simple as your intention, like *Make of My Home a Haven*. Take out all but the first letters of the main words: *MMHH*. And then—here's the fun part—take out a paper and pencil and create a beautiful image that incorporates those letters, but in an obscure and artistic way as in the sigil candle shown here.

You can use charcoal, calligraphy, watercolors—whichever medium feels best for you. Add crosses, embellishments, arrows, swoops—you want to obscure the meaning *and* make it beautiful.

Once you've finished with your first creation, make some others. Make a sigil for peace, for empowerment, for love—and then put them all away. Leave them somewhere you can't see them for a month or so, until the precise meaning of each sigil is forgotten.

When the month has passed, you'll need to charge your sigil—pick just one at a time. This requires reaching a state that is the opposite of what we are usually trying to achieve: you do not want to be mindful; you want to be *mindless*. You want to lose yourself entirely, so that the sigil can take on its own life and power. You are the best judge of the most effective way to shut off your brain, to lose your awareness of self. Dancing like no one is watching? Spinning until you're dizzy? Running until you're so tired all you want to do is lie on the ground, panting? Do whatever works for you.

When you reach that state, focus on your sigil. Hold its image firmly in your mind. Don't imbue it with anything, just give it your still reflection.

And now, you can do what you like with it. If it's beautiful to you, you can hang it in your home. You can burn it to release it. You can make it into a tattoo. Its power is already at work in the world.

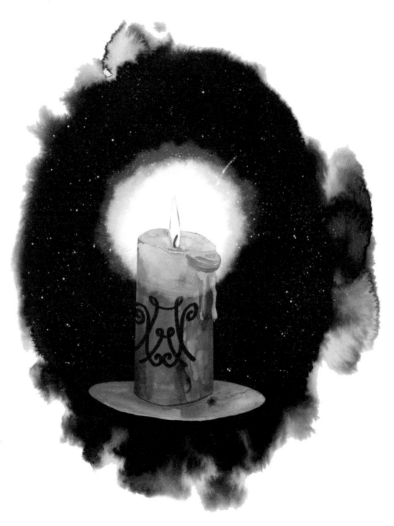

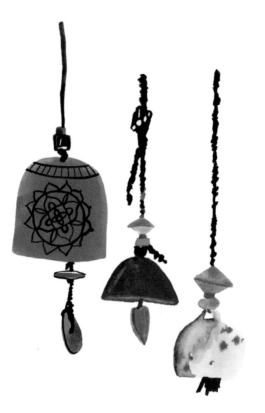

BELLS FOR YOUR DOOR

THE TINKLING OF A BELL AT A DOOR SERVES A LARGER PURPOSE
than letting a store owner know that a customer has arrived. The tone and vibra-
tion invite a clearing, a wave of new energy—which is what happens whenever
we come and go. Hanging the traditional witches' bells on the front door does
act as a sort of early alert system, but it also reminds us to step in and out of our
homes with a sense of freshness, release, and adventure.

Any set of bells with a sound you enjoy will do, but you can also create
your own!

Oven-bake clay like Sculpey
or Fimo

Paint or gloss for oven-bake
clay (optional)

Thin hemp cord

Small or medium-size
craft bells

Start by molding your clay into a bell shape. One block should be enough for one large bell or two smaller bells. They do not need to be perfect! Rounded, square, or a little wiggly—this is creative expression! As you work with the clay, and as you create your shapes and designs, work in your intentions, which will then come through in the vibrations of the bells.

Smooth out your seams, and use a pencil, knife, or your fingernail to add etchings, sigils, or designs onto your bells. Make a hole in the center of each bell. Bake them according to the manufacturer's instructions and allow them to cool completely. Use paint to add stripes or other designs if you like.

When your paint is dry, cut about twelve inches' worth of cord and knot one end of it onto your craft bell. Draw the cord through your clay bell.

Hang them just over your door.

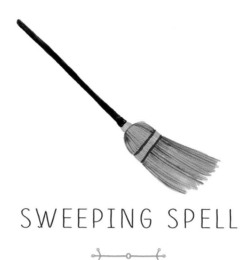

SWEEPING SPELL

SWEEPING CAN BE A MISERABLE TASK, MOSTLY BECAUSE IT tends to feel somewhat pointless—it seems as though the moment we've swept, we sit down to eat and crumbs fall on the floor again, or dirt is tracked in, or the cat sheds, or dust blows in from an open window. And that is always true, because we all continue to *live* in our homes, making them forever not-spotless.

But there is also something deeply satisfying about sweeping, about the sheer amount of *stuff* that fills a dustpan, about the feel of a clean floor beneath bare feet. Sweeping is such a simple act—and such a powerful one. After all, what is more valuable to a witch than her broom?

To connect with the power of sweeping—and avoid thinking of it as another pointless chore—work, as always, with intention. Begin at the outside edges of the room and work clockwise, sweeping ever toward the center. Vary between long smooth strokes and quick heavy brushes. Any negative energy that might be lingering in your house will be gathered up with the dust. When you've finally collected your pile in the center of the room, wave your palm over it, banishing any unwelcome energy you may have collected. Then—throw it away.

If you drop your broom, or angle it against the wall in such a way that it slides to the floor with a clatter, make a wish before picking it up. You never know what will come!

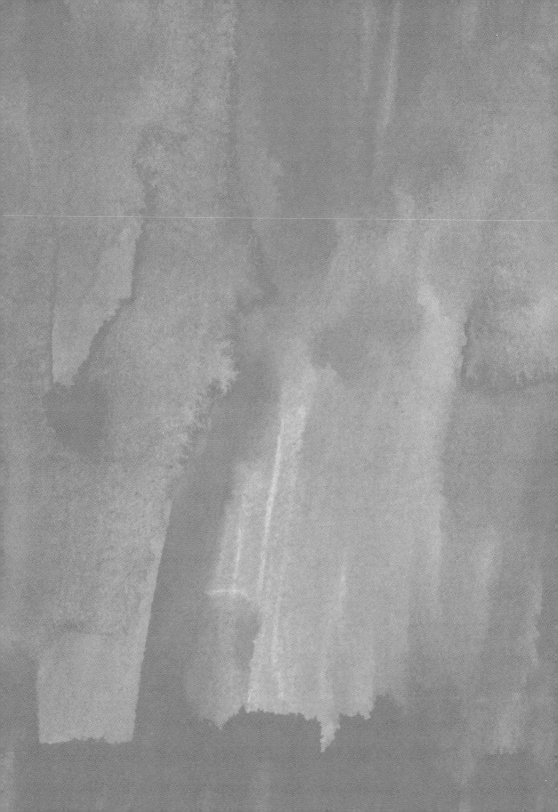

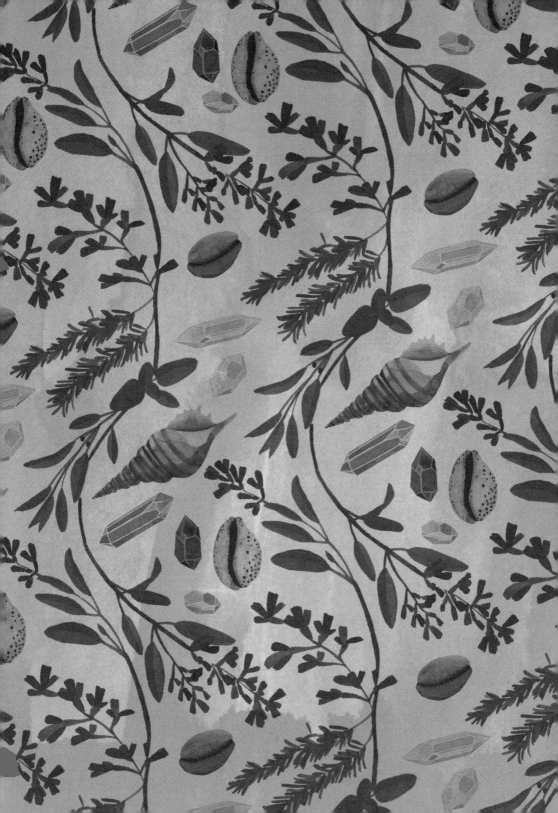

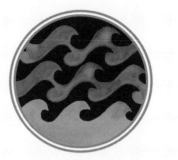

SOOTHING

CRYSTAL GRID

WHILE A CRYSTAL ON ITS OWN IS POWERFUL, ITS ENERGY IS magnified exponentially when connected with vibrancy of others in an intentional geometrical pattern, like a mandala. Crystal grids can be created for any purpose—to invite prosperity, love, or anything you want to create in your life. This grid will welcome peace and purification into your home.

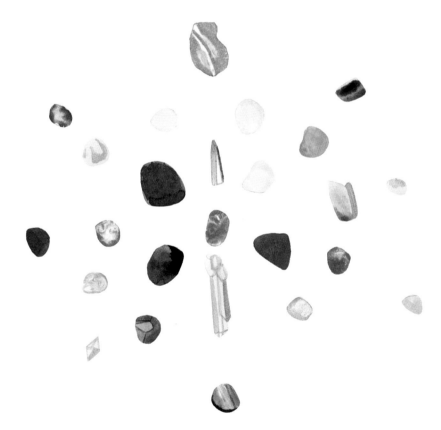

Clear quartz

Hematite

Moonstone

Obsidian

Pyrite

Smoky quartz

You can use any combination of these stones, but you will need between eighteen and thirty-six total. It's useful, for geometrical and magical purposes, to work in multiples of three. You will need one quartz point, as well.

There are crystal grid mats or printouts available, but it's much more creative—and therefore more powerful—to arrange your crystals by sight and feel. The goal is to develop a balanced grid, so vary the black and white colors of your crystals, rather than grouping them all together. If you have some that are wand-shaped rather than rounded, place them in opposition to each other. Aesthetics matter here.

When your grid is complete, take a moment to activate it. Starting from the outside and working your way in toward the center, use your quartz point to draw lines connecting each crystal and bringing them into alignment with each other. Once your grid is activated, leave it in place for at least a full day and night. You can meditate over it during this time, or simply leave it be to do its work—but give it the space and time to do so.

CHARM FOR
RESTFUL SLEEP

WE NEED SLEEP TO SURVIVE, AND YET IT IS ELUSIVE. INSOMNIA is a fact of life for as many as one in three people today, while we are kept awake by our fears, our anxieties, our long list of things left undone. This rumination solves nothing, as a lack of rest makes us only more anxious and less able to complete what we need to do—but the cycle repeats itself night after night.

In addition to your Tylenol PM or your melatonin, try creating this gris-gris bag and placing it beside your pillow at night. You can fall asleep while holding it, or simply keep it close to your head so you can breathe in its scent and feel its power to soothe and relax you.

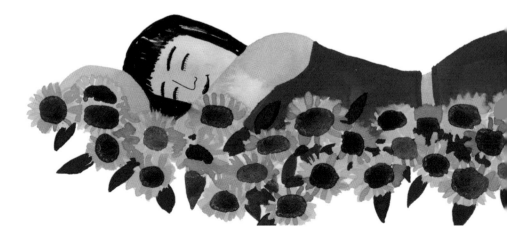

1 tablespoon dried lavender

1 tablespoon dried vervain

1 tablespoon dried yarrow

1 tablespoon dried lemon balm or catnip

Amethyst, for a gentle and restful sleep

You can adjust your gris-gris charm according to your needs: add some holly if you'd like to invite prophetic dreams, cowslip if you would like to be visited by loved ones who have passed, or betony if you require protection from nightmares. You can use angelite to help your brain work through problems while you sleep, labradorite to give your dreams power, hematite to ward off nightmares, or black tourmaline for a deep sleep.

Stir your herbs together and let them charge in the full moon, surrounded by your chosen crystal or crystals. Burn some sage over them if desired, just to be sure you have warded off anything that might want to keep you awake. Gather everything into a small cloth bag and place it lovingly at your side as you prepare for sleep. Change it out every full moon, as needed.

WIND CHIMES

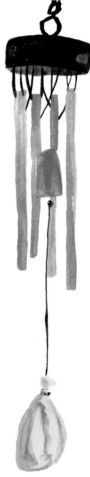

THE AIR THAT FLOWS IN AND AROUND THE HOME BRINGS ALL manner of good, cleansing energy with it. But, of course, since we can't see it, we tend to forget about it. Wind chimes that rock gently in the breeze can be the perfect reminder of the refreshing winds of change.

But you don't want just any wind chimes. The sounds yours makes should evoke something deep within you, that brings a smile whenever you hear it, and that's not really something you can find at a big-box store.

Start with a collection of objects. You want a mix of things—shells, driftwood, mysterious keys that don't seem to open any of your doors, pretty beads, parts of broken necklaces, or the remaining half of a lost pair of earrings. Add anything that you've kept in a drawer even though it has no purpose, just because it speaks to you.

Then look for something to serve as the top of your wind chimes. It can be a piece of wood, an embroidery hoop, or even a big tin can. Select the kind of material you want to use to hang your items—you can use fishing line, twine, leather cording, or thin chains. You can attach your objects to your lines (and your lines to your top) with superglue, hot glue, or even by knotting them in place, depending on what materials you are working with. Arrange your items with several on each strand, or with all of them dangling freely.

Hang your wind chimes where you can see as well as hear them—and smile.

DIY DIFFUSER

꘎——o——꘎

AROMATHERAPY FOR THE HOME IS ABOUT AS IMPORTANT AS any single form of self-care. Scent is the most powerful of our five senses, and it can instantly evoke whatever mood or flavor of magic you're seeking. This recipe is for a soothing, restful scent to reduce your stress levels, but you can easily use myrrh and frankincense to invite psychic power, or rosemary, thyme, and sweet orange to keep you focused and energetic. And it's ridiculously easy.

Glass bottle or jar with a narrow opening

⅓ cup unscented carrier oil, like almond or grapeseed oil

1 tablespoon isopropyl alcohol

10 drops lavender essential oil

10 drops chamomile essential oil

10 drops rose essential oil

3–6 rattan reeds (available at craft stores)

Add your carrier oil to the glass bottle and thin it with the isopropyl alcohol. Add your essential oils and place the reeds in the bottle, stirring the liquid slightly. Allow an hour or two for the oils to move up through the reeds, at which point the scent will last for days or weeks.

PROTECTION SPELL

WHETHER YOU LIVE ON A FIFTY-ACRE FARM OR IN A TINY STUDIO apartment, your home has boundaries, and those boundaries are permeable. We do our best to keep unwanted visitors out with NO TRESPASSING notices, NO SOLICITATIONS stickers, and sturdy locks and fences, but what about visitations that are a bit less solid? A fence can't keep negative energies away, and ill wishes don't care so much about our signage.

Most boundary spells begin with salt, and depending on the length of your perimeter, you may need a lot, though you'll be sprinkling only a few grains at a time.

Start by blessing and clearing your salt. You'll want non-iodized salt, if possible. Fill a bowl and place clear quartz and hematite around it. Leave it in a place where the sun and moon will shine upon it for twenty-four hours.

When you're ready, begin to walk your boundary, sprinkling the salt as you go. Call on any protective spirits, ancestors, or deities you feel you can rely on for safeguarding and aid. If you are working outdoors, do the same at the corners of your property. If you are working indoors, make sure you sprinkle a little extra at your doors and windows, whispering a few words of protection as you do so. You can say something along the lines of:

I call upon [names of spirits, ancestors or deities]
Shield, Bless, Protect
Shield, Bless, Protect

You can create your own spell, simply whisper "protect," or say nothing at all and allow your intentions to speak for you.

You will of course be tempted to sweep up after, especially indoors, but resist the urge for a full twenty-four hours. When the time comes, begin by clearing your windows, then sweep from the outside in toward the center of your home. Whisper your thanks to the salt before you dispose of it.

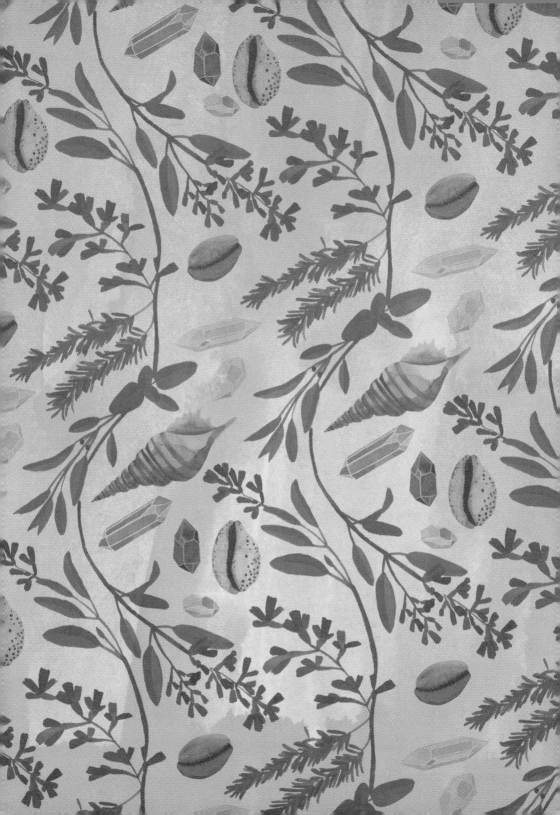

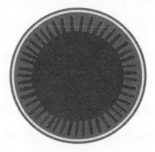

EMPOWERING

ALTAR

EVERY WELLNESS WITCH SHOULD HAVE AN ALTAR. IT SERVES AS A place to focus her thoughts, prepare for meditation or spellwork, and keep her home in the state of soft, resonant power that it should have. But each altar is personal to that witch, and it will change as she changes and as her practice changes.

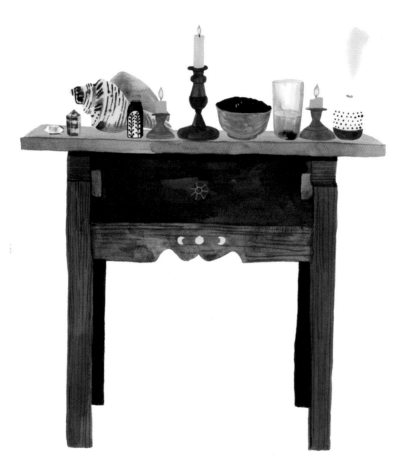

Here are some things to consider, just to get started: You'll want to keep your altar in a somewhat out-of-the-way place, to avoid unwanted questions—if that's a risk—and also to keep others from messing with it. Your altar is yours alone, and it is private. Many witches keep them in a corner of the bedroom or on a dresser or bookshelf. This is a sacred space, but it doesn't have to take up a lot of room.

You may want to incorporate the elements, so consider the following symbols:

FIRE	AIR	WATER	EARTH
Candle	Feather	Seashell	Bowl of loam
Volcanic stones	Diffuser	Empty cup	Horn or bone
Spices like cinnamon or pepper	Wind chimes	Jar of rainwater	Sedimentary rock

You'll also want a central symbol for your altar, perhaps an image or figure of a deity or loved one, a pentagram, a powerful crystal, an incense burner, a bowl, or a chalice—your central symbol will change as you and your needs do.

Those are the basics—the flair is up to you. Enhance your altar with any stones or essential oils that speak to you and any found items like lost keys, shells, driftwood, or bits of string—many altars look like a magpie has been at them, and that's a *good* thing. You'll want to refresh your altar on the changing of the seasons by reflecting on what still feels true and right to you and what needs to be put away for another day.

INCENSE

INCENSE IS POWERFUL, HEADY STUFF—AND CAN SOMETIMES
be overwhelming. A little goes a long way, but it can be incredibly effective in
heightening meditative states and clearing energy.

This isn't that kind of incense. It's not a stick that you light or anything like
that—this is the kind of incense you use to cast over an open flame to invite
visions or prophecy. Gather a combination of the following:

- Dried eyebright
- Dried marigold
- Dried vervain
- Dried hyssop
- Dried mugwort
- Dried wormwood
- Dried lavender
- Dried St. John's wort
- Dried yarrow

If you'll be working over an open fire, you'll want two to four tablespoons total. If
you're working over a candle, you'll want only about a half a teaspoon.

Begin by grinding your herbs in a mortar and pestle until they are as powdery as
you can make them. Place the herbs in a bowl on the night of either the full moon or
the dark of the moon, depending on the kind of vision you seek—if you seek a clearer
understanding of a situation that seems impenetrable, allow the full moon to work
her magic. Or if you simply want to go deep and explore what might be so hidden
you don't even know it's there, let the darkness of the new moon bring you into her
depths. Surround the bowl with amethysts, calcite, lapis lazuli, and opal.

Before attempting to induce your visions, prepare yourself. Wash your hands
and face in cool clear water. Perform a grounding ritual. If you're working over an
open fire, make sure it is safely contained. If you're working over a candle, make
sure it, too, is not a safety risk. Before sprinkling your incense over the flame, protect yourself with hematite, obsidian, pyrite, smoky quartz, and tigereye.

You *may* experience full-on visions, but these herbs are not hallucinogenic,
so it's unlikely. Instead, listen to your voice within, and pay attention to your
dreams. What is your intuition telling you?

RUNES

RUNES, OR FUTHARK, ARE AN ANCIENT GERMANIC SYSTEM OF writing and were also used for divination, protection, and other forms of magic. The word *rune* in fact translates to "holding a secret," as runes were believed to be deeply powerful and could only be understood fully by the wisest and most courageous of people.

Today, runes are often carved onto stones or tiles, which are then carried to keep their magic close or cast as an oracle reading. They are of course available for purchase, but as always, the most powerful magical objects are the ones you make for yourself.

There are twenty-four runes in the Elder Futhark, and they can be combined to create deeper, more complex meanings:

FEHU

Abundance, luck, energy, sexual attraction

URUZ

Health, endurance, determination

THURISAZ

Chaos, destruction, masculine energy

ANSUZ

Order, language, intelligence, communication

RAIDHO

Adventure, leadership, moral responsibility, movement

KENAZ

Knowledge, creativity, craftsmanship

GEBO

Trade, balance,
generosity, gratitude

WUNJO

Joy, contentment,
harmony

HAGALAZ

Crisis, catastrophe,
fate

NAUTHIZ

Resistance, work,
necessity, life lessons

ISA

Stillness, concentration,
but also stagnation

JERA

Harvest, seasons,
fertility, peace

EIHWAZ

Wisdom, ancient
knowledge, mysteries of
life and death

PERTHRO

Fate, luck, prophecy

ALGIZ

Protection, connection
with the gods

SOWILO

The soul, wholeness, confidence

TIWAZ

Justice, sacrifice

BERKANO

Secrecy, fertility, feminine power, healing

EHWAZ

Harmony, cooperation, friendship

MANNAZ

The rational mind, intellect, the human condition

LAGUZ

Water, life, dreams, imagination, emotion

INGUZ

Personal growth, earth, solitude

DAGAZ

The link between twilight and the dawn, awakening, paradox

OTHALA

Household, family, ancestry

So, to create a charm for creativity, you could combine Kenaz and Laguz, like so:

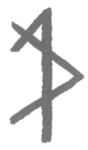

Or you could combine Uruz, Jera, Wunjo, and Ehwaz for a rune of peace and happiness:

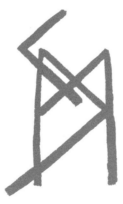

To make your own runic stones, gather twenty-four (or more, in case you want extras if there are any errors!) smooth, rounded stones. You can use river stones, quartz, beach stones—whatever is accessible and feels right to you. Give your stones a good scrubbing with soap and hot water and then allow them to dry completely. Wipe them down with rubbing alcohol to make sure they're completely free of dirt. Using a permanent marker, draw one rune on each of the stones. You'll want to use a black marker for lighter stones and a gold or white marker for darker stones.

Allow your stones to dry for twenty-four hours, in a place where both the sunlight and the moonlight will shine over them. Line a baking sheet with foil, and bake them at 200 degrees for about thirty minutes. Return them to their drying place, and allow them to rest and charge for another twenty-four hours before using.

Rune-casting can be a complex process, and if you want to go deeper into this form of internal divination, there is much to explore. But historically, rune-casting was very simple. To get started, you'll need a white cloth. Sit down and meditate with the question you are asking of the runes. Hold them in their bag, close to your heart. When you are ready to cast, reach into the bag and pull out a handful of stones—it doesn't matter how many, as the correct number will find their way into your fingers. Cast them onto your white cloth.

Any runes that have landed upside down (i.e., you can't read them), set aside. You'll focus only on the runes that are face-up. Now, take your time. What runes do you see? How do they lie in relation to each other? Two that are close together are likely intertwined in meaning. Runes are often read left-to-right in terms of timeline, so that runes to the left represent something in the past, while runes to the center represent the present, and runes to the right tell of the future.

This is very open to personal interpretation. As you and your runes get to know each other, you will devise ways to communicate.

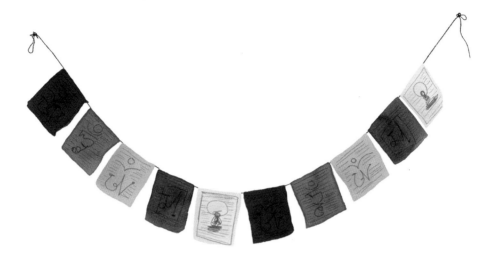

DIY PRAYER FLAGS

TIBETAN PRAYER FLAGS ARE COLORED RECTANGULAR CLOTHS, frequently strung on a line like bunting. They are traditionally used to bless the surrounding countryside or home, inviting peace, compassion, and wisdom. They don't exactly carry prayers to the gods, but instead the winds spread the goodwill of the flags to all who are nearby.

They are lovely, and if Bon or Tibetan Buddhism is part of your practice, then the traditional flags of these religions make a wonderful addition to your home. But you can also take inspiration from this tradition and create your own, using whatever method best appeals to you.

You'll need about a yard of white cotton or linen fabric, some sharp scissors, and a needle and thread. Cut the fabric into six-by-nine-inch rectangles. There's no need to hem or otherwise finish the fabric—a little fraying is part of the aesthetic. Fold the top of the rectangle down by half an inch (you can iron it to keep it straight) and stitch it down, creating a tube for the flag to hang by. Make as many as you like, depending on where you want to hang them.

And now ask yourself, what kind of magic do I want to use to imbue my flags with my prayers and intentions? Do you want to use thread magic and embroider sigils, runes, or inspirational quotes or spells? Or do you want to use the power of nature, and paint with fabric paint on leaves and ferns to create stamps for your flags? You can use stencils or hand-quilting. You can even purchase printable fabric to hang some of your favorite images or quotes. Embellish your images with buttons or ribbons as desired, incorporating the colors of the chakras.

Thread some yarn or cord through your flags, tying knots at each end of each flag to keep them evenly spaced. And then hang them in a spot where the wind will blow through them and carry your well-wishes into your greater community.

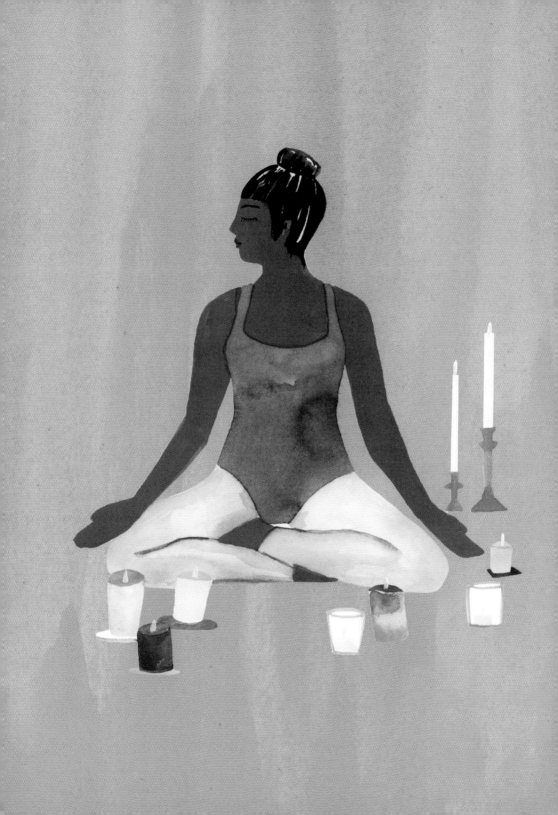

CANDLE SPELL

CANDLE SPELLS HAVE BEEN AROUND FOR ABOUT AS LONG AS
there have been candles, as the allure of the hypnotic power of fire likely dates
back to its very discovery. You can use any candle for this, but a purple, frankin-
cense-scented candle is particularly effective, as it draws on both the power of
the sun and your crown chakra. If you can't find one with this color or scent, you
can easily make this candle by adapting the White Sandalwood Candle (see
page 97).

Set yourself up by finding a comfortable seat, either on a chair or a meditation pillow or simply on the floor, and place your candle on a shelf or low table
so that it is right at eye height—you don't want to strain your neck by looking up
or down for too long. If this isn't feasible, but you're comfortable sitting on the
floor, you can place the candle on the floor three to six feet away from you—this
is where the gaze falls naturally, and so shouldn't be harmful.

Do this practice at night or with the shades lowered, so that the light is
dim. Take three long, deep breaths, inhaling as much as you can and exhal-
ing as much as you can. Allow your gaze to soften as you stare at the flame.
Watch it dance.

Focus on the flame, and imbue it with meaning. Give it power, and take
power from it. The fire is destruction; you have the ability to destroy that which
blocks you. The fire is warmth; you have warmth and compassion to give and to
receive. The fire is passion; it stokes the flame within you. The fire is life; you live
with the vibrancy and unfettered joy of the dancing flame.

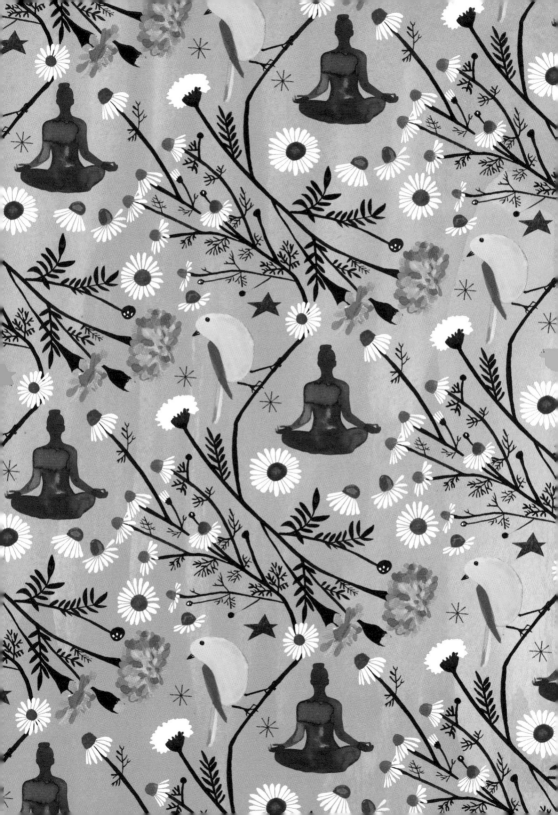

CONCLUSION

As you continue your journey through the practice and lifestyle of wellness magic, consider this book as a jumping-off point. If there is any single takeaway from the practices we've explored here, it's that magic is not something you *learn,* but something you do and create, by and for yourself.

Magic is personal, and it responds differently to each of us—as we respond differently to magic. You may have found a certain connection to particular crystals or that they responded differently to you than indicated here. You may have found an affinity for certain herbs or for certain kinds of spellwork, while others didn't feel quite right. This is not only to be expected; it's deeply important! It is our own individual connection to our work that matters.

Take that information and extrapolate from it. If the tactile nature of crafting magic appeals to you, follow that path and see where it leads you. If the purity and efficacy of herbal magic are more your jam, there is a whole wide world of herbalism waiting to be explored. If the mystery, intention, and ritual of meditative magic call to you, then seeking a deeper mystical understanding will be a great adventure.

Enjoy the journey.

ACKnOWLeDGMenTS

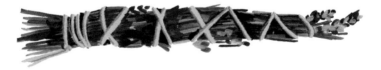

Maile, I couldn't have written this book without you.
You are my fellow witch, always, and thank you so much for your help. Dave,
I promise I'll make some more granola bars at some point. Mom and Dad,
thank you for recipe testing and Mabon celebrations—Dad, you got a real
acknowledgment this time!

Shannon Connors Fabricant, witch-sister and "make it magical" inspiration, thank you always. Susan Van Horn and Anisa Makhoul, thank you so
much for making this book so beautiful. Ashley Benning, thank you for check-
ing my verb-switches! Kristin Kiser, thank you for this next adventure.

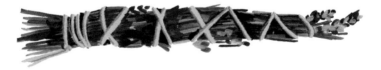

Index

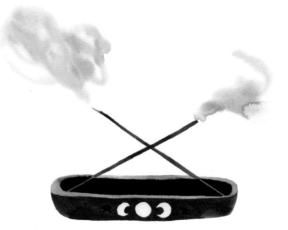